Roberto Patarca-Montero, MD, PhD
Editor

Innovations in Chronic Fatigue Syndrome Research and Clinical Practice

Innovations in Chronic Fatigue Syndrome Research and Clinical Practice has been co-published simultaneously as *Journal of Chronic Fatigue Syndrome*, Volume 8, Numbers 3/4 2001.

Pre-publication REVIEWS, COMMENTARIES, EVALUATIONS . . .

"This volume helps to bring CFS into the mainstream, a definable illness with known sociology, demographics and even treatment. It will bring light to a previously murky topic."

Ethan Russo, MD
Neurologist
Author of Handbook of Psychotropic Herb

Innovations
in Chronic Fatigue Syndrome
Research and Clinical Practice

Innovations in Chronic Fatigue Syndrome Research and Clinical Practice has been co-published simultaneously as *Journal of Chronic Fatigue Syndrome*, Volume 8, Numbers 3/4 2001.

<u>The *Journal of Chronic Fatigue Syndrome* Monographic "Separates"</u>

Below is a list of "separates," which in serials librarianship means a special issue simultaneously published as a special journal issue or double-issue *and* as a "separate" hardbound monograph. (This is a format which we also call a "DocuSerial.")

"Separates" are published because specialized libraries or professionals may wish to purchase a specific thematic issue by itself in a format which can be separately cataloged and shelved, as opposed to purchasing the journal on an on-going basis. Faculty members may also more easily consider a "separate" for classroom adoption.

"Separates" are carefully classified separately with the major book jobbers so that the journal tie-in can be noted on new book order slips to avoid duplicate purchasing.

You may wish to visit Haworth's website at . . .

http://www.HaworthPress.com

. . . to search our online catalog for complete tables of contents of these separates and related publications.

You may also call 1-800-HAWORTH (outside US/Canada: 607-722-5857), or Fax 1-800-895-0582 (outside US/Canada: 607-771-0012), or e-mail at:

getinfo@haworthpressinc.com

Innovations in Chronic Fatigue Syndrome Research and Clinical Practice, edited by Roberto Patarca-Montero, MD, PhD (Vol. 8, No. 3/4, 2001). *"WILL BRING LIGHT TO A PREVIOUSLY MURKY TOPIC. . . . Helps bring CFS into the mainstream: a definable illness with known sociology, demographics, and even treatment." (Ethan Russo, MD, Neurologist; Author, Handbook of Psychotropic Herbs)*

Chronic Fatigue Syndrome: Critical Reviews and Clinical Advances, edited by Kenny De Meirleir, MD, and Roberto Patarca-Montero, MD, PhD (Vol. 6, No. 3/4, 2000). *The reviews in this volume provide the specialized views of different schools of thought, research, and clinical intervention for CFS and ME (myalgic encephalomyelitis). Edited by the organizer of the Second World Congress on Chronic Fatigue Syndrome and Related Disorders, this work focuses on information gathered there. Keep your knowledge of these disorders and current and up-to-date with Chronic Fatigue Syndrome: Critical Reviews and Clinical Advances!*

Chronic Fatigue Syndrome: Advances in Epidemiologic, Clinical, and Basic Science Research, edited by Roberto Patarca-Montero, MD, PhD (Vol. 5, No. 3/4, 1999). *Highlights the presentations and issues discussed at the recent Fourth Annual International Conference of the American Association of Chronic Fatigue Syndrome (CFS). You will explore the strengths and weaknesses of current case definitions of CFS and how these can be improved. Also, you will examine how to distinguish CFS from other similar ailments such as fibromyalgia and multiple chemical sensitivity. This book puts different therapeutic modalities to the test, and addresses the neurological and psychiatric manifestations associated with CFS.*

Disability and Chronic Fatigue Syndrome: Clinical, Legal and Patient Perspectives, edited by Nancy G. Klimas, MD, and Roberto Patarca, MD, PhD (Vol. 3, No. 4, 1997). *"As a physician who deals with disability issues daily, I found this volume fascinating and informative. This is 'must read' material for anyone involved with the disability process and CFS." (Charles W. Lapp, MD, Director, Hunter-Hopkins Center, Charlotte, North Carolina)*

Clinical Management of Chronic Fatigue Syndrome: Clinical Conference, American Association of Chronic Fatigue Syndrome, edited by Nancy Klimas, MD, and Roberto Patarca, MD, PhD (Vol. 1, No. 3/4, 1995). *"A truly interdisciplinary approach to the investigation and management of a debilitating and complex disorder." (The Annals of Pharmacotherapy)*

Innovations
in Chronic Fatigue Syndrome
Research and Clinical Practice

Roberto Patarca-Montero, MD, PhD
Editor

Innovations in Chronic Fatigue Syndrome Research and Clinical Practice has been co-published simultaneously as *Journal of Chronic Fatigue Syndrome*, Volume 8, Numbers 3/4 2001.

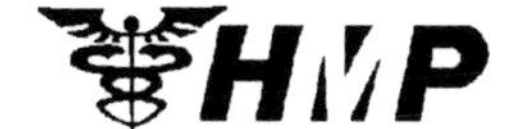

The Haworth Medical Press
An Imprint of
The Haworth Press, Inc.
New York • London • Oxford

Published by

The Haworth Medical Press®, 10 Alice Street, Binghamton, NY 13904-1580 USA

The Haworth Medical Press® is an imprint of The Haworth Press, Inc., 10 Alice Street, Binghamton, NY 13904-1580 USA.

Innovations in Chronic Fatigue Syndrome Research and Clinical Practice has been co-published simultaneously as *Journal of Chronic Fatigue Syndrome*, Volume 8, Numbers 3/4 2001.

Cover design by Thomas J. Mayshock Jr.

Library of Congress Cataloging-in-Publication Data

Innovations in chronic fatigue syndrome research and clinical practice/Roberto Patarca-Montero, editor.
     p. cm.
    This text "has been co-published simultaneously as Journal of chronic fatigue syndrome, volume 8, numbers 3/4 2001."
    Includes bibliographical references and index.
    ISBN 0-7890-1425-4 (hard: alk. paper)–ISBN 0-7890-1426-2 (pbk.: alk. paper)
    1. Chronic fatigue syndrom. I. Patarca-Montero, Roberto.

RB150.F37 I565 2001
616'.0478–dc21
                                        2001039493

Indexing, Abstracting & Website/Internet Coverage

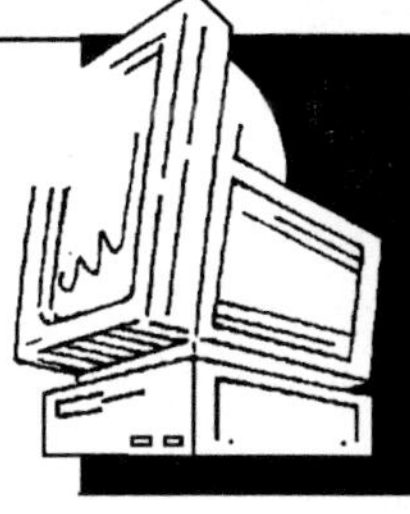

This section provides you with a list of major indexing & abstracting services. That is to say, each service began covering this periodical during the year noted in the right column. Most Websites which are listed below have indicated that they will either post, disseminate, compile, archive, cite or alert their own Website users with research-based content from this work. (This list is as current as the copyright date of this publication.)

Abstracting, Website/Indexing Coverage . . . . Year When Coverage Began

- *Abstracts in Anthropology*. **1995**

- *AIDS Abstracts* **1995**

- *Behavioral Medicine Abstracts* **1996**

- *BUBL Information Service, an Internet-Based Information
  Service for the UK higher education community,
  <URL: http://bubl.ac.uk/>* **1995**

- *Centre Regional d'Exploration des Myalgias
  <http://www.infomyalgie.com>* **1998**

- *CFS-NEWS* **1999**

- *CINAHL (Cumulative Index to Nursing & Allied Health
  Literature)* **1995**

- *CNPIEC Reference Guide: Chinese National Directory
  of Foreign Periodicals* **1995**

- *EMBASE/Excerpta Medica Secondary Publishing Division
  <URL: http://www.elsevier.nl>*. **1995**

(continued)

(continued)

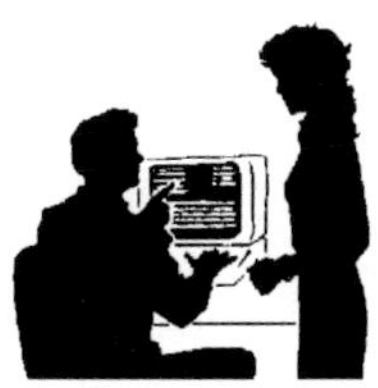

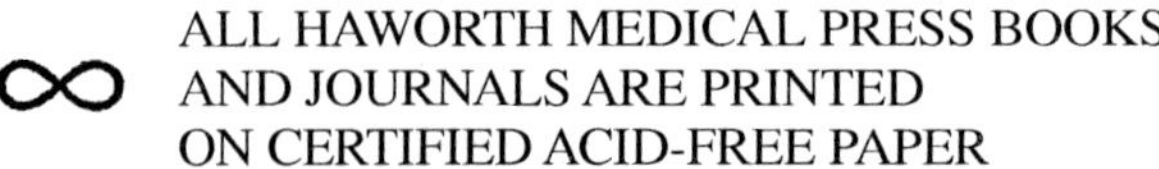

Innovations in Chronic Fatigue Syndrome Research and Clinical Practice

CONTENTS

ABOUT THE EDITOR

Roberto Patarca-Montero, MD, PhD, is Assistant Professor of Microbiology and Immunology and also serves as Co-Director of the E.M. Papper Laboratory of Clinical Immunology at the University of Miami, School of Medicine. Previously, he was Assistant Professor of Pathology at the Dana-Farber Cancer Institute and Harvard Medical School in Boston. Dr. Patarca-Montero was a member of the Board of Directors of the American Association for Chronic Fatigue Syndrome. Dr. Patarca-Montero also served as editor of *Critical Reviews in Oncogenesis* and is the author or co-author of more than 100 articles in journals or books. He is currently conducting research on immunotherapy in AIDS.

Preface

The V International Meeting of the American Association for Chronic Fatigue Syndrome in Seattle, Washington brought together patients, healthcare professionals, and researchers in a well-structured forum. This volume includes articles that cover material presented and discussed at the meeting. The first set of articles pertain to studies that are part of the efforts to refine the research and clinical definition of CFS and to agree on a new name for the disease. The name controversy is not trivial because, as documented in the articles in this issue and voiced repeatedly by patients and many healthcare professionals, the misnomer of CFS has a negative impact in many areas. The second set of articles in this puplication deals with pathophysiology and treatment. The advent of the post-genomics era is also evident in the field of CFS research as elegantly exemplified by the articles by Roelens et al. and Englebienne et al. These articles together with the presentation by Dr. Paul Cheney's group on the presence of particular Alu repeat-derived nucleic acid fragments in the sera of CFS patients are opening the door for the definition of markers that have the potential not only to serve as the basis for diagnosis and/or follow-up assays but also to explain the multiple manifestations of CFS. Novel therapies can also be designed with these new targets in mind. The job in hand now is to document the reliability (sensitivity and specificity across a wide spectrum of diseases) and universality (among CFS patients) of the markers presented. Other interesting material presented at the meeting, for instance the abnormalities in sympathetic tone in CFS patients and its consequences including rhinitis, have been published in previous issues of *Journal of Chronic Fatigue Syndrome*.

Roberto Patarca-Montero, MD, PhD

[Haworth co-indexing entry note]: "Preface." Patarca-Montero, Roberto. Co-published simultaneously in *Journal of Chronic Fatigue Syndrome* (The Haworth Medical Press, an imprint of The Haworth Press, Inc.) Vol. 8, No. 3/4, 2001, p. xvii; and: *Innovations in Chronic Fatigue Syndrome Research and Clinical Practice* (ed: Roberto Patarca-Montero) The Haworth Medical Press, an imprint of The Haworth Press, Inc., 2001, p. xiii. Single or multiple copies of this article are available for a fee from The Haworth Document Delivery Service [1-800-342-9678, 9:00 a.m. - 5:00 p.m. (EST). E-mail address: getinfo@haworthpressinc.com].

     xiii

Subtypes of Chronic Fatigue Syndrome:
A Review of Findings

Leonard A. Jason, PhD
Renée R. Taylor, PhD
Cara L. Kennedy, BA
Susan Torres Harding, MA
Sharon Song, MA
Danielle Johnson, BA
Radhika Chimata, BA

SUMMARY. Most studies of Chronic Fatigue Syndrome (CFS) have been based on patients recruited from primary or tertiary care settings.

Leonard A. Jason, Renée R. Taylor, Cara L. Kennedy, Susan Torres Harding, Sharon Song, Danielle Johnson, and Radhika Chimata are affiliated with the Department of Psychology, DePaul University.

Address correspondence to: Leonard A. Jason, Department of Psychology, DePaul University, 2219 North Kenmore Avenue, Chicago, IL 60614.

Financial support for this study was provided by NIAID grant number AI36295.

[Haworth co-indexing entry note]: "Subtypes of Chronic Fatigue Syndrome: A Review of Findings." Jason, Leonard A. et al. Co-published simultaneously in *Journal of Chronic Fatigue Syndrome* (The Haworth Medical Press, an imprint of The Haworth Press, Inc.) Vol. 8, No. 3/4, 2001, pp. 1-21; and: *Innovations in Chronic Fatigue Syndrome Research and Clinical Practice* (ed: Roberto Patarca-Montero) The Haworth Medical Press, an imprint of The Haworth Press, Inc., 2001, pp. 1-21. Single or multiple copies of this article are available for a fee from The Haworth Document Delivery Service [1-800-342-9678, 9:00 a.m. - 5:00 p.m. (EST). E-mail address: getinfo@haworthpressinc.com].

Patients from such settings might not be typical of patients in the general population and may not accurately reflect the heterogeneity among individuals diagnosed with this condition. The current paper reviews four community-based studies that examined subtypes of individuals with CFS. Distinctions between subtype groups based on sociodemographics, illness onset and duration, stressful precipitating events, symptom frequency, and comorbidity characteristics are made with respect to outcome measures of fatigue and symptom severity, functional ability, and psychiatric comorbidity. *[Article copies available for a fee from The Haworth Document Delivery Service: 1-800-342-9678. E-mail address: <getinfo@ haworthpressinc.com> Website: <http://www.HaworthPress.com> © 2001 by The Haworth Press, Inc. All rights reserved.]*

KEYWORDS. CFS definition, symptomatology, population studies

Chronic Fatigue Syndrome (CFS) is a highly heterogeneous condition, affecting different people in different ways, and fluctuating in terms of symptoms and severity during illness course (Anderson & Ferrans, 1997). It can affect virtually every major system in the body; neurological, immunological, hormonal, gastrointestinal and musculoskeletal problems have been reported (Friedberg & Jason, 1998). One major challenge facing CFS research is the issue of patient heterogeneity. Across studies, individuals with CFS have been found to differ with respect to characteristics such as gender, ethnicity, and socioeconomic status, mode of illness onset and duration of illness, symptom severity, functional disability, psychiatric comorbidity, and coping styles (Friedberg & Jason, 1998). As a result of this heterogeneity, findings emerging from studies in a number of areas are, at best, discrepant, and at worst, contradictory, and the field has become highly polarized with respect to issues involving etiology, diagnosis, epidemiology, and treatment. Uncontrolled patient heterogeneity in empirical studies is one consequence of ignoring this important issue of sub-classification. When unique patient groups are unwittingly combined, any distinctions pertaining to specific subtypes of CFS become blurred.

For years, investigators have noted many biological abnormalities among patients with CFS, including over-activated immune systems (Landay, Jessop, Lennette, & Levy, 1991), biochemical dysregulation in the 2-5A synthetase/RNase L pathway (Suhadolnik et al., 1997), cardiac dysfunction (Lerner, Lawrie, & Dworkin, 1993), EEG abnormalities (Donati, Fagioli, Komaroff, & Duffy, 1994), abnormalities in cerebral white matter (Natelson, Cohen, Brassloff, & Lee, 1993), decreases in blood flow in certain areas of the brain (Schwartz et al., 1994), and autonomic nervous system dysfunction (Freeman & Komaroff, 1997). However, there has been a lack of consistency in such laboratory findings, which may be a function of combining distinctive groups of patients into a large heterogeneous group rather than analyzing them within subtypes.

Recent studies illustrate that sociodemographic variables can play an important role in highlighting key distinctions between individuals with CFS surrounding illness severity and functional disability. Several studies have highlighted commonalities among individuals with CFS, including greater likelihood of being female, Caucasian, and of higher socioeconomic status (Reyes et al., 1997; Gunn, Connell, & Randall, 1993). However, community-based studies involving representative samples of ethnically and socioeconomically diverse populations indicate that the prevalence of CFS is actually higher for minority groups of Latinos and African-Americans than for Caucasians (Jason, Richman et al., 1999), and higher for individuals of lower socioeconomic status than for those of higher socioeconomic status (Wessely, Chalder, Hirsch, Wallace, & Wright, 1997). CFS continues to be found to be more prevalent among women than men (Jason, Richman et al., 1999), and there is some evidence to indicate that there are gender-related differences in the impact of CFS as well as in prevalence. Among a sample of individuals with CFS, women were found to have a higher frequency of fibromyalgia, tender/enlarged lymph nodes, and lower scores on the physical functioning subscale of the MOS, while men had higher frequency of pharyngeal inflammation and a higher lifetime prevalence of alcoholism (Buchwald, Pearlman, Kith, & Schmaling, 1994). It is important for investigators to more frequently examine sociodemographic subtype differences like these in patients with CFS.

Findings from many empirical investigations of CFS suggest that subtypes of patients can be also distinguished with respect to the mode of illness onset (whether gradual or sudden) (DeLuca, Johnson, Ellis, & Natelson, 1997; Reyes et al., 1999; Komaroff, 1988, 1994; Levine, 1997), the presence of a stressful life event preceding or precipitating onset of CFS (Ray, Jeffries, & Weir; 1995; Salit, 1997; Theorell, Blomkvist, Lindh, & Evengard, 1999), and the duration of the illness. Reyes and associates (1999), examined symptoms experienced at illness onset for individuals with either sudden or gradual onset of CFS. Those with sudden onset reported significantly more symptoms at onset than those with gradual onset, and symptoms were more likely to be of infectious nature, including fever, sore throat, chills, and tender lymph nodes. This is consistent with other research (Komaroff, 1988, 1994) suggesting that sudden onset of CFS may be indicative of viral or other infectious illness. Some evidence indicates that individuals with CFS have experienced a higher frequency of negative life events in the time directly preceding the onset than matched controls (Salit, 1997; Theorell et al., 1999). With respect to duration of illness, some researchers (Clark et al., 1995; Ray, Jeffries, & Weir, 1997) have determined that persistent illness and poorer outcomes could be predicted by longer duration of CFS symptoms. Wilson and associates (1994), however, did not find duration of illness to be a predictor of outcome, and Hill, Tiersky, Scavalla, and Natelson (1999) found that neither duration of illness nor mode of onset predicted illness outcome. Clearly, more research is needed to examine these important subtypes.

Findings suggest that patients with CFS can also be distinguished in terms of symptom frequency and severity. In a US sample, Manu and associates (1988) found a bimodal distribution of symptoms among 100 chronic fatigue patients, including 21 patients with 10-15 symptoms and 79 patients with 0-9 symptoms. In two follow-up studies of patients with CFS, persistent symptoms and disability at the follow-up were associated with having eight or more medically unexplained symptoms at initial evaluation (Clark et al., 1995; Bombardier & Buchwald, 1995). A comparison group of non-CFS chronic fatigue patients exhibited fewer symptoms and higher functioning (Bombardier & Buchwald, 1995). It seems apparent that patients with a higher number of symptoms are more functionally impaired than those with fewer symptoms.

Many of the symptoms associated with CFS are also characteristic of Fibromyalgia (FM). In the absence of definitive diagnostic markers or laboratory tests to distinguish these conditions, clinical diagnosis is largely based on self-report symptoms and behavioral criteria. Several previous studies have suggested that CFS and FM have many similarities (Buchwald, 1996; Goldenberg, 1988; Goldenberg, Simms, Geiger & Komaroff, 1990), although rates of comorbidity between CFS and FM are highly disparate. Another subtype that would be useful to investigate in future studies involves comparing those patients with only CFS versus those patients with CFS and FM.

In addition to comorbidity of medical illnesses such as FM with CFS, debate exists with respect to the issue of psychiatric comorbidity among individuals with CFS, and the research community is polarized as to the role of psychiatric illness in the etiology, course, and progress of CFS. Some researchers (Gold et al., 1990; Katon, Buchwald, Simon, Russo,

& Mease, 1991; Manu, Lane, and Matthews, 1988; Taerk, Toner, Salit, Garfinkel, & Ozersky, 1987) have found psychiatric illness to play a primary role in development and course of CFS, while others (Hickie, Lloyd, Wakefield, & Parker, 1990; Yeomans & Conway, 1991; Stone et al., 1994) have provided evidence against such findings. Comparing patients with psychiatric comorbidity versus those without psychiatric comorbidity involves another important area of subtyping for CFS research.

Findings from a community-based epidemiologic study of CFS have examined several distinctive subtype groups of individuals with CFS, including subtypes based on sociodemographic variables (Jason et al., 2000a), variables related to illness onset and duration (Jason et al., 2000b), symptom frequency (Jason et al., 2001a), and comorbidity with other illness, including fibromyalgia and psychiatric illness (Jason et al., 2001b). This article reviews and summarizes results of these studies, and highlights the implications of subtype findings for future research.

METHOD

The data derive from a larger community-based study of CFS (see Jason, Jordan et al., 1999; Jason, Richman et al., 1999 for details), which was carried out in three stages. Stage 1 entailed a cross-sectional screening telephone survey of a random sample of 28,673 adults, with 18,675 adults completing the screening interview. Stage 2 involved a structured psychiatric interview for those respondents from Stage 1 who screened positive for CFS (i.e., six or more months of fatigue, and at least four minor symptoms based on the Fukuda et al., 1994, criteria). Stage 3 involved a medical exam and structured medical history for the same group of participants agreeing to undergo further evaluation.

Design and Statistical Analyses

Measures

Screening Questionnaire. The Stage 1 screening questionnaire assessed interviewees' sociodemographic characteristics and preliminary classification into screened positive (CFS-like) versus screened negative groups. This screening questionnaire has been found to have adequate reliability (Jason, Ropacki et al., 1997). Basic demographic data included age, ethnicity, socioeconomic status, marital status, and gender. The revised scoring rules for Hollingshead's (1975) scale, developed and validated by Wasser (1991), were used to classify socioeconomic status. These encompassed explicit definitions of occupation and education.

Psychiatric Interview. In Stage 2, the Structured Clinical Interview for the DSM-IV (SCID) (Spitzer, Williams, Gibbon, & First, 1995) was used to assess exclusionary and non-exclusionary current and lifetime psychiatric diagnoses as defined on Axis I of the Diagnostic and Statistical Manual of Mental Disorders-Fourth Edition (DSM-IV) (American Psychiatric Association, 1994). As such, it served two purposes in the present study. First, it was administered to all CFS-like and control participants undergoing evaluation to rule out exclusionary psychiatric illnesses that could explain fatigue symptomatology. Once a subgroup of individuals with CFS was diagnosed and identified as having no exclusionary conditions, the SCID was then used as an outcome measure to measure subtype differences in rates of non-exclusionary psychiatric conditions (current and lifetime). The SCID is a valid and reliable semi-structured interview guide that approximates a traditional psychiatric interview (Rubinson & Asnis, 1989). Trained advanced clinical psychology graduate students with master's degrees administered the SCID.

Physician Examination: A physician conducted a detailed medical examination to rule out exclusionary medical conditions and detect evidence of diffuse adenopathy, hepatosplenomegaly, synovitis, neuropathy, myopathy, cardiac or pulmonary dysfunction, or any other medical disorder. An 18-tender-point examination was used to test for fibromyalgia (Goodnick & Sandoval, 1993). Laboratory tests administered to all participants included a chemistry screen (glucose, calcium, electrolytes, uric acid, liver function tests, and renal function tests), complete blood count with differential and platelet count, T4 and TSH, erythrocyte sedimentation rate, arthritic profile (which included rheumatoid factor and antinuclear antibody), hepatitis B surface antigen, CPK, HIV screen and urinalysis.

Diagnosis: A team of four physicians and a psychiatrist were responsible for making final CFS diagnoses. Two physicians independently rated each file using the current U.S. definitions of CFS (Fukuda et al., 1994) and FM (Wolfe et al., 1990). If a disagreement occurred, a third physician rater was used. Individuals were diagnosed with concurrent Fibromyalgia if they met the current case definition (Wolfe et al., 1990).

Outcome Measures

Symptom Severity. Participants were also asked to complete the CFS Symptom Rating Form. Using this form, participants rated the severity of the eight CFS definitional symptoms (Fukuda et al., 1994). Social/recreational activities were rated on a 10-point scale, with 0 = normal levels before the illness, 5 = half of one's normal level, and 10 = activities completely curtailed. Work activities were also rated on a 10-point scale, with 0 = full-time work without any difficulty, 5 = half of one's normal level, and 10 = not able to work at all. In a previous study (Jason, Ropacki et al., 1997), a modified version of this form was demonstrated to have high test-retest reliability over a two-week period (test-retest agreement: 76%-92%).

Medical Outcomes Study. Patients also completed the Medical Outcomes Study 36-Item Short-Form Survey (Ware & Sherbourne, 1992), a reliable and valid measure that discriminates between gradations of disability. This instrument encompasses eight multi-item scales that assess physical functioning, physical role limitations, bodily pain, general health perceptions, vitality, social functioning, emotional role functioning, and mental health, with higher scores indicating a better health status. For each participant, raw scores were converted to scaled scores and scaled scores were then summed for each of the eight MOS functional domains according to guidelines provided in the MOS scoring manual (Medical Outcomes Trust, 1994). Overall, higher scaled score totals indicate better health or less functional impairment. The MOS has demonstrated adequate psychometric properties as a measure of functional status in a population of individuals with CFS, and it has distinguished CFS from other fatiguing illnesses (Buchwald et al., 1996).

Cope Scales. The Cope scales (Carver, Scheier, & Weintraub, 1989) were used to measure the following types of coping strategies: Seeking Emotional Social Support; Positive Reinterpretation and Growth; Acceptance; Denial; Turning to Religion; Behavioral Disengagement; and Focusing on and Venting Emotions. Respondents were asked to rate these items based upon what they thought about when they were under a lot of stress. Each of the subscales has scores ranging from 4-16, with higher scores indicating more use of that particular coping strategy. This is a well-validated instrument that has adequate reliability (Carver et al., 1989).

Illness Management Questionnaire. The Illness Management Questionnaire (IMQ) (Ray, Weir, Stewart, Miller, & Hyde, 1993) was developed specifically to assess coping in patients with CFS, and has been used extensively in studies of adults with CFS (Ray, Jeffries, & Weir, 1995). The IMQ has four factors: Maintaining Activity (attempting to ignore symptoms, disregarding possible adverse effects of activity); Accommodating to the Illness (organizing and arranging one's life to avoid exertion and manage stress); Focusing on Symptoms (preoccupation with symptoms, how one views the extent over which the illness dominates one's life); and Information Seeking (searching for relevant information and an openness to trying treatments). The instrument provides a measure of problem-focused coping, rather than one that is focused on the management of distress. The time period assessed by this instrument is for the past month. Test-retest reliabilities of the IMQ range from .85 (Information Seeking) to .93 (Maintaining Activity). Higher scores on the IMQ indicate greater use of each coping style.

Life Orientation Test. The revised version of the Life Orientation Test (LOT) (Scheier & Carver, 1985) was used as a measure of cognitive appraisals for an overall score of Optimism. Respondents are asked to indicate whether they currently agreed or disagreed (based on a five point scale) with each of 13 items (some items are fillers). This well-validated scale has a total score that ranges from 0-24, with higher scores indicating more optimism.

Perceived Stress Scale. The Perceived Stress Scale (PSS), is a four-item revised version of a previous 14-item measure of global perceived stress. The time period that this instrument measured was the last month (Cohen, Kamarck, & Mermelstein, 1983). The authors report a coefficient alpha reliability of .72 for the four-item short version. The Total Stress score ranges from 0-16, with higher scores reflecting more stress.

RESULTS AND DISCUSSION

Sociodemographics

In the first of the reviewed studies (Jason et al., 2000a), important differences emerged between subtypes of individuals with CFS based on sociodemographic variables of gender, ethnicity and work status. An examination of gender differences revealed that women were less likely to be working full-time, reported significantly more impairment in work activities, were more likely to have children, and were more likely to have greater numbers of children than men. Women also had significantly poorer physical functioning, more bodily pain, poorer emotional role functioning, and significantly more severe muscle pain. In part, the experience of more severe symptomatology and functional disability among women with CFS may serve as an explanation for why they comprised 100% of the non-working group. Previous findings for significantly better physical functioning in men with CFS (Buchwald, Pearlman, Kith, & Schmaling, 1994) provide some support for these results. Increased symptom severity and poorer functional outcomes among women may involve certain predisposing vulnerabilities that may be more likely to occur in women than in men, such as biological factors involving reproductive correlates (Harlow, Signorello, Hall, Dailey, & Komaroff, 1998) and biopsychosocial factors such as stress-associated immune modulation (Glaser & Kiecolt-Glaser, 1998).

Women in comparison to men were also found to have greater perceived stress. It is not clear whether this stress may have been associated, in part, with evidence for increased child rearing responsibilities reported among women in this sample. However, a study of quality of life of individuals with CFS (Anderson & Ferrans, 1997), found that more women than men felt that CFS had negatively impacted their family life, with more women expressing shame, guilt, or sadness over increasing dependency on family members. This unique form of illness-related stress experienced by women may, in part, account for the differences both in illness severity and perceived stress found in the Jason et al. (2000a) study.

Women not only perceived greater degrees of stress, but they were also more likely to turn to religion as an emotion-focused coping style (Jason et al., 2000a). Results from other studies of coping among women with chronic illnesses support this finding. One study comparing coping styles in HIV-infected and non-infected women (Biggar et al., 1999) found that infected women were more likely to use religion (prayer) as a coping mechanism. In another study, women with arthritis were also more likely to turn to religion or prayer as a method of coping (Abraido-Lanza, Guir, & Revenson, 1996). A third study comparing coping in women and men with memory aging also found that women scored significantly higher than men on use of religiosity as a coping strategy (McDougall, 1998).

In addition to sociodemographic differences related to gender, ethnic group differences were also explored (Jason et al., 2000a). Findings indicated that individuals classified as minorities experienced significantly more severe symptomatology including sore throats, postexertional malaise, headaches, and unrefreshing sleep than Caucasians, and they reported poorer general health status. CFS is not only more prevalent among minority populations (Jason, Richman et al., 1999), but results from this reviewed study also reveal that the symptoms are experienced more acutely in minority populations (Jason et al., 2000a). These findings may partly be explained by the interaction of factors contributing to poorer health status among underserved ethnic groups, including psychosocial stress, behavioral risk factors (use of alcohol and tobacco and lack of sufficient exercise), differences in health care practices (inadequate nutrition and lack of routine medical examinations), barriers to access to adequate health care (lack of health insurance and inadequate health care), and more hazardous occupations and environmental exposures (Davis, 1995; Perez-Stable, Marin & VanOss-Marin, 1994; Ruiz, 1995).

Differences also emerged in the coping styles of minorities and Caucasians, with minorities being significantly more likely to turn to religion, use denial, and use behavioral disengagement as means of coping (Jason et al., 2000a). Findings regarding use of religion as a coping mechanism among minorities are supported by Abraido-Lanza, Guir, and Revenson (1996) who found that in a sample of 109 Latinas of low socioeconomic status with arthritis, the use of religion or prayer was the second most commonly reported coping strategy. Abraido-Lanza and associates attributed this coping response to culture-based notions of coping as well as culturally valued norms such as familism. In a study of Black and White Americans (Millet, Sullivan, Schwebel, & Myers, 1996), Black Americans were also found to rate spiritual factors as more important in the etiology and treatment of difficulties than did White Americans.

Findings from the reviewed study of sociodemographic factors also highlight the potential value of using work status as a guide for identifying low- and high-functioning subgroups of individuals with CFS (Jason et al., 2000a). Results indicated that working individuals reported less severe muscle and joint pain and better physical functioning than their non-working counterparts. Working CFS participants also reported higher occupational, social, and recreational activity levels, and were less likely to use the coping mechanism of positive reinterpretation/growth than non-working CFS participants (possibly because they were more satisfied with their current occupational and social circumstances).

In summary, findings demonstrate that sociodemographic heterogeneity among individuals with CFS can account for significant differences in the CFS illness experience. Characteristics such as gender, ethnicity, and work status were found to be related to differences in illness severity, functional outcomes, coping styles, and perceived stress, but unrelated to differences in psychiatric comorbidity.

Mode of Onset, Stressful Events, and Illness Duration

A second study by Jason and associates (2000b) revealed symptomatic and functional differences related to mode of onset, presence of stressful events, and illness duration. Findings for increased sore throat severity and more severe fatigue following exercise, in conjunction with a directional tendency toward higher psychiatric comorbidity in the sudden onset group, may provide support for defining a subgroup of patients characterized by an increased likelihood of viral or infectious illness. Schwartz and associates (1994) found neurological defects in a sample of individuals with CFS that explained sudden-onset, flu-like symptoms of CFS and depression, which may have been linked to chronic viral encephalitis.

In investigating whether stressful life events preceded or precipitated CFS onset, findings from the reviewed study (Jason et al., 2000b) indicated that half of the individuals with CFS in the present study were able to identify a stressful event occurring at the time of onset. This proportion is lower than that estimated by prior research that has found a clear association between psychosocial factors and CFS onset (Salit, 1997; Theorell et al., 1999). In particular, Salit (1997) found that stressful events were common in the year preceding CFS onset (occurring in 85% of the sample). Similarly, Theorell and associates (1999) found that individuals with CFS were nearly twice as likely to report the occurrence of negative life events during the three months preceding onset. Possible explanations for the differences between rates of occurrence of stressful life events in the reviewed study and prior studies may be due to differences in timing criteria for the stressful event. Prior studies have targeted occurrence during the preceding one year (Salit, 1997) or the preceding three months (Theorell et al., 1999), while the reviewed study targeted events occurring directly at the time of onset.

In comparing individuals who were able to identify unusually severe stress associated with CFS onset to those who were unable to identify any particular stressful event, significant differences emerged on the vitality and emotional role functioning scales of the MOS (Jason et al., 2000b). Individuals who were experiencing unusually severe stress at the time of onset reported lower levels of vitality and lower emotional role functioning. Stresses reported by these individuals included family problems, death of a loved one, marital separation, financial difficulty, and medical problems. One potential explanation for the differences in vitality and emotional role functioning may involve enduring emotional stress from these events, which may continue to deplete feelings of energy and interfere with work or other daily activities. Additionally, these differences may be linked to the work of Ray and associates (1995), that found negative life-events to be associated with higher anxiety. Individuals who have experienced stressful life events at onset that continue to produce anxiety may consequently suffer diminished vitality and impaired emotional functioning.

With respect to duration of illness, individuals with shorter duration of illness reported better general health on the MOS, indicating that they perceived their health as better and had a more optimistic outlook regarding recovery than those with longer illness duration (Jason et al., 2000b). In contrast to these differences in overall perceptions of health, however, analyses of outcome measures revealed that the severity of most CFS symptoms (with the exception of lymph node pain, which was significantly more severe among individuals with shorter duration of illness) remained stable throughout the course of the illness, regardless of duration. Taken together, these two findings may indicate that individuals with shorter illness duration, though just as ill as those with longer duration, are more likely to be optimistic about overall self-perceived health and prognosis. This suggests that although self-perceived illness severity may change based on illness duration, symptom severity is less likely to change significantly according to illness duration. Self-perceived illness severity may, in part, be subject to differences with respect to duration of illness because those with shorter duration may be using denial as a means of coping with the onset of a new and debilitating illness. In support of this explanation, an empirical examination of the psychosocial phases of the CFS illness using members of the CFIDS Association (a national self-help organization) indicated that individuals with shortest illness duration were more likely to use denial of illness chronicity and expectation of a cure as means of coping with the illness (Jason, Fennell et al., 2000). In contrast to findings of stable symptom severity over time, however, Joyce, Hotopf, and Wessely (1997) have reported a decline in symptom severity and frequency over time. One possible explanation for this discrepancy may involve differences in the constructs measured (e.g., symptoms versus perceived overall health). Present findings indicate that the psychological effects of illness may change over time, leaving individuals with a more pessimistic outlook regarding their health and prognosis than when they first became ill.

The second reviewed article (Jason et al., 2000b) revealed symptomatic and functional differences across mode of onset, presence of stressful events, and illness duration. These findings point to a need for further research on viral etiology and symptomatology, the connection between symptom severity and perception of severity over time, and causal factors precipitating illness.

High versus Low Symptom Frequency

The sample of individuals with CFS in the third reviewed study (Jason et al., 2001a) was divided into two subgroups: those who experienced a high frequency of symptoms rated at a severity of 40 or higher on a 100-point scale versus those who experienced a low frequency of symptoms at a severity of 40 or higher. In defining subtypes of low versus high frequency, 0-100 ratings for each of 66 cognitive and somatic symptoms (including the eight CFS definitional symptoms; Fukuda et al., 1994) were required to meet a predetermined threshold of severity (rating of 40 or higher) to be considered at a rate considered as at least moderate to high. Low frequency was determined as 0-13 symptoms, and high frequency was determined as 14 or more. When subtypes were determined in this manner, differences emerged with respect to gender, age, work status, and functional disability. All individuals experiencing high symptom frequency were female, and all male participants in this sample experienced low symptom frequency. Symptom frequency impacted individuals' ability to work and maintain functional abilities. Those with high frequency were older, less likely to be working full-time, more likely to be unemployed, on disability, or working part-time, and more functionally disabled according to MOS subscales of physical functioning, physical role functioning, bodily pain, and emotional role functioning.

Contrary to the findings of prior studies (Hickie et al., 1995; Manu et al., 1988), psychiatric status in the reviewed study (Jason et al., 2001a) did not vary significantly according to subtyping of individuals based on symptom frequency. These findings stand in contrast to those of Hickie et al. (1995), who determined that one distinctive subtype of individuals with CFS included those with greater frequency of CFS and atypical symptoms, greater disability attributed to CFS, and more psychiatric symptoms. Findings in the Jason et al. (2001a) study may indicate that there are actually fewer differences between subtypes of patient groups with respect to psychiatric comorbidity than prior research has suggested.

While the current case definition for CFS (Fukuda et al., 1994) requires that four or more minor symptoms accompany persistent fatigue, the reviewed study (Jason et al., 2001a) demonstrates that some individuals with CFS may experience a great number of other medical symptoms. Results indicate that the presence or absence of such additional symptoms influences individuals' functional ability, and that there may actually be two subgroups of people with CFS: those who experience a large number of additional medical symptoms and those who do not. It is possible that those experiencing a large number of additional symptoms may have comorbid medical illnesses that contribute to observations of increased symptomatology.

Comorbidity

In comparing individuals with CFS and comorbid FM to those with CFS only, results of the reviewed study (Jason et al., 2001b) indicate that comorbidity with FM is associated with an increase in CFS symptom severity and functional impairment. Individuals with both CFS and FM reported significantly less physical functioning, more bodily pain, more severe sore throat pain, muscle pain, and joint pain, more severe fatigue following exercise, more memory/concentration impairment, and more impairment of work activities than individuals without comorbid FM. The findings are consistent with a study (Bombardier & Buchwald, 1996) that found that patients diagnosed with both CFS and FM were substantially more disabled than patients with either condition alone. The presence of greater symptom severity and impairment in individuals diagnosed with both CFS and FM suggests that the two illnesses are not identical, and that CFS and FM present with different types and levels of symptomatology. It is possible that there are underlying systemic differences between individuals with CFS only and those with CFS and FM that are associated with greater overall illness severity and more functional impairment in the latter group. Given that there were no significant differences between these two subgroups in terms of psychiatric comorbidity, stress, and coping, differences in symptomatology appear to be independent of psychiatric and psychosocial status.

Jason and associates (2001b) determined that approximately half of the individuals with CFS reported the presence of a premorbid psychiatric diagnosis. The absence or occurrence of psychiatric illness prior to CFS onset was unrelated to sociodemographic variables, measures of fatigue and symptom severity, disability, stress, and coping. The absence of findings for differences in outcome between those with and without a premorbid diagnosis suggests that a history of psychiatric illness alone does not suffice as an etiological explanation for CFS. Findings from the reviewed study (Jason et al., 2001b) are consistent with those of prior researchers (Hickie, Lloyd, Wakefield, & Parker, 1990; Lloyd, Hickie, Boughton, Spencer, & Wakefield, 1990) who have found no evidence for increased rates of premorbid psychiatric diagnoses among individuals with CFS as compared to community estimates. Prior findings have also suggested that the presence of psychiatric symptomatology among individuals with CFS is likely to be a consequence of, rather than an antecedent risk factor to CFS (Hickie et al., 1990), possibly resulting from the functional limitations and debilitating symptomatology related to CFS. Other research (Kreusi, Dale, & Straus, 1989; DeLuca, Johnson, Ellis, & Natelson, 1997; Wessely, Chalder, Hirsch, Wallace, & Wright, 1996), however, has found CFS to be associated with measures of premorbid psychiatric diagnoses.

With respect to current psychiatric diagnoses (e.g., active at time of interview), rates of comorbidity determined in the present study fall within the middle range (55%) of previous estimates (2.0%-76.5%) (Taylor & Jason, 1998). Analysis of sociodemographic differences revealed that individuals from the CFS sample in the reviewed study (Jason et al., 2001b) who had current psychiatric diagnoses were more likely to have children than those without current psychiatric diagnoses. With respect to outcome measures, individuals with current psychiatric diagnoses demonstrated more overall fatigue and had more impaired emotional role functioning (indicating the interference of emotional problems with ability to spend time on and accomplish occupational or other daily activities). Findings for impaired emotional role functioning are consistent with results from a prior study (Wagner-Raphael, Jason, & Ferrari, 1999), that indicated impaired emotional role functioning among a sample of nurses with CFS who also had current psychiatric disorders. These findings suggest that individuals with comorbid psychiatric disorders perceive their fatigue as more severe and experience greater difficulty with occupational functioning, pointing to a need for more intense and comprehensive forms of intervention for this subgroup of individuals with CFS.

In terms of lifetime psychiatric diagnoses (e.g., including those active at time of interview, those occurring after CFS onset but resolved prior to interview, and those occurring prior to CFS onset), approximately eighty percent of the individuals with CFS in this community-based sample reported having been diagnosed with a psychiatric illness at some point in their lives (Jason et al., 2001b). Although rates of psychiatric comorbidity tend to vary across studies, this finding is consistent with the upper range of prior reports (Katon & Walker, 1993). Individuals with comorbid lifetime psychiatric diagnoses exhibited higher physical fatigue, more severe sore throats, poorer emotional role functioning, greater difficulty accommodating to the illness, and greater levels of perceived stress than those without comorbid lifetime diagnoses. These results indicated that individuals with lifetime psychiatric diagnoses reported that their emotional problems interfered with their ability to spend time working carefully and accomplishing occupational or other daily activities, and that they experienced more difficulty organizing and planning their lives in order to avoid overexertion and control stress. Results also suggested that this patient subgroup felt more overwhelmed by and less confident in their ability to manage stress. Taken together, these findings suggest that individuals with comorbid lifetime psychiatric illness experience more overall stress and have more difficulty coping with emotional challenge and symptoms associated with CFS, and general tasks of daily living.

In summary, findings from this review demonstrate that sociodemographic and illness heterogeneity among individuals with CFS can account for significant differences in the CFS illness experience. Characteristics such as gender, ethnicity, work status, type of illness onset and duration, and illness comorbidity were found to be related to differences in illness severity, functional outcomes, coping styles, and perceived stress, but unrelated to differences in psychiatric comorbidity. Subtype differences detected herein may account for some of the inconsistencies in findings across prior studies that have grouped patients with CFS into one category. Future research which serves to delineate subgroups of patients within the CFS population may result in more consistent findings across studies, which can then be used to more appropriately and sensitively treat the wide range of illness experiences reported by different groups of individuals with CFS.

REFERENCES

Abraido-Lanza, A.F., Guir, C., & Revenson, T.A. (1996). Coping and social support resources among Latinas with arthritis. *Arthritis Care Research, 9* (6), 501-508.

American Psychiatric Association (1994). *Diagnostic and statistical manual of mental disorders* (4th ed.). Washington, DC: Author; 1994.

Anderson, J.S., & Ferrans, C.E. (1997). The quality of life of persons with chronic fatigue syndrome. *The Journal of Nervous and Mental Disease, 185* (6), 359-367.

Barsky, A.J. & Borus, J.F. (1999). Functional somatic syndromes. *Annals of Internal Medicine, 130*, 910-921.

Biggar, H., Forehand, R., Devine, D., Brody, G., Armistead, L., Morse, E., & Simon, P. (1999). Women who are HIV infected: The role of religious activity in psychosocial adjustment. *AIDS Care, 11* (2), 195-199.

Bombardier, C.H. & Buchwald, D. (1995). Outcome and prognosis of patients with chronic fatigue syndrome. *Archives of Internal Medicine, 155*, 2105-2110.

Bombardier, C.H. & Buchwald, D. (1996). Chronic fatigue, chronic fatigue syndrome, and fibromyalgia: Disability and health care use. *Medical Care, 34*, 924-930.

Buchwald, D. (1996). Fibromyalgia and chronic fatigue syndrome: Similarities and differences. *Rheumatic Diseases Clinics of North America, 22*, 219-243.

Buchwald, D. & Garrity, D. (1994). Comparison of patients with chronic fatigue syndrome, fibromyalgia, and chemical sensitivities. *Archives of Internal Medicine, 154*, 2049-2053.

Buchwald, D., Pearlman, T., Kith, P., & Schmaling, K. (1994). Gender differences in patients with chronic fatigue syndrome. *Journal of General Internal Medicine, 9*, 387-401

Buchwald, D., Pearlman, T., Umali, J., Schmaling, K., & Katon, W. (1996). Functional status in patients with chronic fatigue syndrome, other fatiguing illnesses, and healthy individuals. *American Journal of Medicine, 101*, 364-370.

Carver, C.S., Scheier, M.F., & Weintraub, J.K. (1989). Assessing coping strategies: A theoretically based approach. *Journal of Personality and Social Psychology, 56* (2), 267-283.

Clark, M.R., Katon, W., Russo, J., Kith, P., Sintay, M., & Buchwald, D. (1995). Chronic fatigue: Risk factors for symptom persistence in a two and one half year followup study. *American Journal of Medicine, 98,* 187-195.

Cohen, S., Kamarck, T., & Mermelstein, R. (1983). A global measure of perceived stress. *Journal of Health and Social Behavior, 37* (2), 147-153.

Davis, R. (1995). Racial differences in mortality: Current trends and perspectives. In (G.E. Thomas, Ed.), *Race and ethnicity in America: Meeting the challenge in the 21st century* (pp. 115-126). Washington, DC: Taylor & Francis.

Deary, I.J. (1999). A taxonomy of medically unexplained symptoms. *Journal of Psychosomatic Research, 47*, 51-59.

DeLuca, J., Johnson, S.K., Ellis, S.P., & Natelson, B.H. (1997) Sudden versus gradual onset of chronic fatigue syndrome differentiates individuals on cognitive and psychiatric measures. *Journal of Psychiatric Research, 31*, 83-90.

Donati, F., Fagioli, L., Komaroff, A.L., & Duffy, F.H. (1994, Oct.). *Quantified EEG Findings in patients with Chronic Fatigue Syndrome.* Paper presented at the American Association of Chronic Fatigue Syndrome Research Conference. Ft. Lauderdale, FL.

Freeman, R., & Komaroff, A.L. (1997). Does the chronic fatigue syndrome involve autonomic nervous system? *American Journal of Medicine, 102*, 357-364.

Friedberg, F., & Jason, L.A. (1998). *Understanding chronic fatigue syndrome: An empirical guide to assessment and treatment.* Washington, DC: American Psychological Association.

Fukuda, K., Straus, S.E., Hickie, I., Sharpe, M.C., Dobbins, J.G., & Komaroff, A. (1994). The Chronic Fatigue Syndrome: A comprehensive approach to its definition and study. *Annals of Internal Medicine, 121,* 953-959.

Glaser, R., & Kiecolt-Glaser, J.K. (1998). Stress-associated immune modulation: Relevance to viral infections and chronic fatigue syndrome. *American Journal of Medicine, 105,* 35-42.

Gold, D., Bowden, R., Sixbey, J., Riggs, R., Katon, W.J., Ashley, R., Obrigewitch, R.M., & Corey, L. (1990). Chronic fatigue. A prospective clinical and virologic study. *Journal of the American Medical Association, 264,* 48-53.

Goldenberg, D.L. (1988). Research in fibromyalgia: Past, present and future. *Journal of Rheumatology, 15,* 992-996.

Goldenberg, D.L., Simms, R.W., Geiger, A., & Komaroff, A.L. (1990). High frequency of fibromyalgia in patients with chronic fatigue seen in a primary care practice. *Arthritis and Rheumatism, 31,* 381-387.

Goodnick, P.J., & Sandoval, R. (1993). Psychotopic treatment of chronic fatigue syndrome and related disorders. *The Journal of Clinical Psychiatry, 51* (1), 13-20.

Gunn, W.J., Connell, D.B., & Randall, B. (1993). Epidemiology of chronic fatigue syndrome: The Centers-for-Disease-Control study. In B.R. Bock & J. Whelan (Eds.), *Chronic Fatigue Syndrome* (pp. 83-101). New York: John Wiley & Sons.

Harlow, B.L., Signorello, L.B., Hall, J.E., Dailey, C., & Komaroff, A.L. (1998). Reproductive correlates of chronic fatigue syndrome. *American Journal of Medicine, 105,* 94S-99S.

Hickie, I., Lloyd, A., Wakefield, D., & Parker, G. (1990). The psychiatric status of patients with chronic fatigue syndrome. *British Journal of Psychiatry 1990, 156,* 534-540.

Hickie, I., Lloyd, A., Wilson, A., Hadzi-Pavlovic, D., Parker, G., Bird, K., & Wakefield, D. (1995). Can the Chronic Fatigue Syndrome be defined by distinct clinical features? *Psychological Medicine, 25,* 925-935.

Hill, N.F., Tiersky, L.A., Scavalla, V.R., & Natelson, B.H. (1999). Fluctuation and outcome of chronic fatigue syndrome over time. *Journal of Chronic Fatigue Syndrome, 5* (3/4), 93-94.

Hollingshead, A.B. (1995). Four factor index of social status. (Unpublished manuscript, available from Department of Sociology, Yale University, New Haven, CT).

Hudson, J.I., Goldenberg, D.L., Pope, H.G., Keck, P.E., & Schlesinger, L. (1992). Comorbidity of fibromyalgia with medical and psychiatric disorders. *American Journal of Medicine, 92,* 363-367.

Jason, L.A., Fennell, P.A., Taylor, R.R., Fricano, G., & Halpert, J.A. (2000). An empirical verification of the Fennell phases of the CFS illness. *Journal of Chronic Fatigue Syndrome, 6,* 47-56.

Jason, L.A., Jordan, K.M., Richman, J.A., Rademaker, A.W., Huang, C., McCready, W., Shlaes, J., King, C.P., Landis, D., Torres, S., Haney-Davis, T., & Frankenberry, E.L. (1999). A community-based study of prolonged and chronic fatigue. *Journal of Health Psychology, 4,* 9-26.

Jason, L.A., Richman, J.A., Rademaker, A.W., Jordan, K.M., Plioplys, A.V., Taylor, R., McCready, W., Huang, C., & Plioplys, S. (1999). A community-based study of chronic fatigue syndrome. *Archives of Internal Medicine, 159,* 2129-2137.

Jason, L.A., Ropacki, M.T., Santoro, N.B., Richman, J.A., Heatherly, W., Taylor, R., Ferrari, J.R., Haney-Davis, T.M., Rademaker, A., Dupuis, J., Golding, J., Plioplys, A.V., Plioplys, S. (1997). A Screening Instrument for Chronic Fatigue Syndrome: Reliability and validity. *Journal of Chronic Fatigue Syndrome, 3*, 39-59.

Jason, L.A., Taylor, R.R., Kennedy, C.L., Jordan, K., Song, S., Johnson, D.E., Torres, S.R. (2000a). Chronic Fatigue Syndrome: Sociodemographic subtypes in a community-based sample. *Evaluation and the Health Professions, 23*, 243-263.

Jason, L.A., Taylor, R.R., Kennedy, C.L., Song, S., Johnson, D.E., & Torres, S.R. (2000b). Chronic fatigue syndrome: Occupation, medical utilization, and subtypes in a community-based sample. *Journal of Nervous and Mental Disease, 188*, 568-576.

Jason, L.A., Taylor, R.R., Kennedy, C.L., Jordan, K., Song, S., Johnson, D.E., & Torres, S.R. (2001a). Chronic fatigue syndrome: Symptom subtypes in a community-based sample. Manuscript submitted for publication

Jason, L.A., Taylor, R.R., Kennedy, C.L., Jordan, K., Song, S., Johnson, D.E., Torres, S.R. (2001b). Chronic fatigue syndrome: Comorbidity with fibromyalgia and psychiatric illness. Manuscript submitted for publication.

Joyce, J., Hotopf, M., & Wessley, S. (1997). The prognosis of chronic fatigue and chronic fatigue syndrome: A systemic review. *Quarterly Journal of Medicine, 90*, 223-233.

Katon, W.J., Buchwald, D.S., Simon, G.E., Russo, J.E., & Mease, P.J. (1991). Psychiatric illness in patients with chronic fatigue and rheumatoid arthritis. *Journal of General Internal Medicine, 6*, 277-285.

Katon, W.J., Walker, E.A. (1993). *The relationship of chronic fatigue to psychiatric illness in community, primary care, and tertiary care samples.* In Bock B.R., Whelan J., editors. *Chronic Fatigue Syndrome.* New York: John Wiley & Sons; pp. 193-211.

Komaroff, A.L. (1988). Chronic fatigue syndromes: Relationship to chronic viral infections. *Journal of Virology Research, 21*, 3-10.

Komaroff, A.L. (1994). Clinical presentation and evaluation of fatigue and chronic fatigue syndrome. In S.E. Straus (Ed.) *Chronic Fatigue Syndrome* (pp. 61-84). New York: Marcel Dekker, Inc.

Kruesi, M.J., Dale, J., & Straus, S.E. (1989). Psychiatric diagnosis in patients who have chronic fatigue syndrome. *Journal of Clinical Psychiatry, 50*, 53-56.

Landay, A.L., Jessop, C., Lennette, E.T., & Levy, J.A. (1991). Chronic fatigue syndrome: Clinical condition associated with immune activation. *The Lancet, 338*, 707-712.

Lerner, A.M., Lawrie, C., & Dworkin, H.S. (1993). Repetitively negative changing T waves at 24-h electrocardiographic monitors in patients with chronic fatigue syndrome. *Chest, 104*, 1417-1421.

Levine, P.H. (1997). Epidemiologic advances in chronic fatigue syndrome. *Journal of Psychiatric Research, 31* (1), 7-18.

Lloyd, A.R., Hickie, I., Boughton, C.R., Spencer, O., & Wakefield, D. (1990). Prevalence of chronic fatigue syndrome in an Australian population. *Medical Journal of Australia 1990, 153*, 522-528.

Manu, P., Lane, T.J., & Matthews, D.A. (1988). The frequency of the Chronic Fatigue Syndrome in patients with symptoms of persistent fatigue. *Annals of Internal Medicine, 109*, 554-556.

McDougall, G.J. (1998). Gender differences in coping and control with memory aging. *Journal of Women and Aging, 10* (1), 21-40.

Medical Outcomes Trust (1994). *How to Score the SF-36 Health Survey*. Boston, MA: Author.

Millet, P.E., Sullivan, B.F., Schwebel, A.I., & Myers, L.J. (1996). Black Americans' and White Americans' views of the etiology and treatment of mental health problems. *Community Mental Health Journal, 32* (3), 235-252.

Natelson, B.H., Cohen, J.M., Brassloff, I., & Lee, H.J. (1993). A controlled study of brain magnetic resonance imaging in patients with fatiguing illnesses. *Journal of the Neurological Sciences, 120*, 213-217.

Perez-Stable, E.J., Marin, G., & VanOss-Marin, B. (1994). Behavioral risk factors: A comparison of Latinos and non-Latino Whites in San Francisco. *American Journal of Public Health, 84*, 971-976.

Ray, C., Jeffries, S., & Weir, W.R. (1997). Coping and other predictors of outcome in chronic fatigue syndrome: A 1-year follow-up. *Journal of Psychosomatic Research, 43* (4), 405-415.

Ray, C., Jeffries, S., & Weir, W.R.C. (1995). Life-events and the course of chronic fatigue syndrome. *British Journal of Medical Psychology, 68*, 323-331.

Ray, C., Weir, W., Stewart, D., Miller, P., & Hyde, G. (1993). Ways of coping with chronic fatigue syndrome: Development of an illness management questionnaire. *Social Science Medicine, 37* (3), 385-391.

Reyes, M., Dobbins, J.G., Nisenbaum, R., Subedar, N.S., Randall, B., & Reeves, W.C. (1999). CFS progression and self-defined recovery: Evidence from the CDC surveillance system. *Journal of Chronic Fatigue Syndrome, 5* (1), 17-27.

Reyes, M., Gary, H.E., Dobbins, J.G., Randall, B., Steele, L., Fukuda, K., Holmes, G.P., Connell, D.G., Mawle, A.C., Schmid, D.S., Stewart, J.A., Schonberger, L.B., Gunn, W.J., & Reeves, W.C. (1997). Surveillance for chronic fatigue syndrome: Four U.S. Cities, September 1989 through August 1993. *Morbidity and Mortality Weekly Report, 46* (SS-2), 1-13.

Rubinson, E.P., & Asnis, G.M. (1989). Use of structured interviews for diagnosis. In S. Wetzler (Ed.), *Measuring Mental Illness: Psychometric assessment for clinicians* (pp. 45-66). Washington, DC: American Psychiatric Press, Inc.

Ruiz, P. (1995). Assessing, diagnosing, and treating culturally diverse individuals: A Hispanic perspective. *Psychiatric Quarterly, 66*, 329-341.

Scheier, M., & Carver, C. (1985). Optimism, coping, and health: Assessment and implications of generalized outcome expectancies. *Health Psychology, 4*, 219-247.

Schwartz, R.B., Komaroff, A.L., Garada, B.M., Gleit, M., Doolittle, T.H., Bates, D.W., Vasile, R.G., & Holman, B.L. (1994). SPECT imaging of the brain: Comparisons of findings in patients with chronic fatigue syndrome, AIDS dementia complex, and major unipolar depression. *American Journal of Radiology, 162*, 943-951.

Salit, I.E. (1997). Precipitating factors for the chronic fatigue syndrome. *Journal of Psychiatric Research, 31* (1), 59-65.

Spitzer, R.L., Williams, J.B.W., Gibbon, M., & First, M.B. (1995). *Structured Clinical Interview for DSM-IV - Non-Patient Edition* (SCID-NP, Version 2.0). Washington DC: American Psychiatric Press; 1995.

Stone, A.A., Broderick, J.E., Porter, L.S., Krupp, L., Gnys, M., Paty, J.S., & Shiffman, S. (1994). Fatigue and mood in Chronic Fatigue Syndrome patients: Results of a momentary assessment protocol examining fatigue and mood levels and diurnal patterns. *Annals of Behavioral Medicine, 16*, 228-234.

Suhadolnik, R.J., Peterson, D.L., O'Brien, K., Cheney, P.R., Hirst, C.V., Reichenbach, N.L., Kon N., Horvath, S.E., Iacono, K.T., Adelson, M.E., DeMeirleir, K., DeBecker, P., Charubula, P., & Pfleiderer, W. (1997). Biochemical evidence for a novel low molecular weight 2-5A-dependent RNase L in chronic fatigue syndrome. *Journal of Interferon and Cytokine Research, 7*, 377-385.

Taerk, G.S., Toner, B.B., Salit, I.E., Garfinkel, P.E., & Ozersky, S. (1987). Depression in patients with neuromyathenia (benign myalgic encephalomyelitis). *International Journal of Psychiatry in Medicine, 17*, 49-56.

Taylor, R.R., & Jason, L.A. (1998). Comparing the DIS with the SCID: Chronic fatigue syndrome and psychiatric comorbidity. *Psychology and Health, 13*, 1087-1104.

Theorell, T., Blomkvist, V., Lindh, G., & Evangard, B. (1999). Critical life events, infections, and symptoms during the year preceding chronic fatigue syndrome (CFS): An examination of CFS patients and subjects with a nonspecific life crisis. *Psychosomatic Medicine, 61* (3), 304-310.

Wagner-Raphael, L.I., Jason, L.A., Ferrari, J.R. (1999). Chronic fatigue syndrome, chronic fatigue, and psychiatric disorders: Predictors of functional status in a national nursing sample. *Journal of Occup Health Psychol, 4*, 63-71.

Wasser, T.E. (1991, August). Statistical correction of Hollingshead's four factor index of social status. Paper presented at the American Psychological Association, San Francisco, CA.

Ware, J.E., & Sherbourne, C.D. (1992). The MOS 36-item Short-Form Health Survey (SF-36): Conceptual framework and item selection. *Medical Care*, June, 473-483.

Wessely, S., Chalder, T., Hirsch, S., Wallace, P., & Wright, D. (1996). Psychological symptoms, somatic symptoms, and psychiatric disorder in chronic fatigue and chronic fatigue syndrome: A prospective study in the primary care setting. *American Journal of Psychiatry, 153*, 1050-1059.

Wessely, S., Chalder, T., Hirsch, S., Wallace, P., & Wright, D. (1997). The prevalence and morbidity of chronic fatigue and chronic fatigue syndrome: A prospective primary care study. *American Journal of Public Health, 87*, 1449-1455.

Wilson, A., Hickie, I., Llyod, A., Hadzi-Pavlovic, D., Boughton, C., Dwyer, J., & Wakefield, D. (1994). Longitudinal study of outcome of chronic fatigue syndrome. *British Medical Journal, 308* (6931), 756-759.

Wolfe, F., Smythe, H.A., Yunus, M.B., Bennett, R.M., Bombardier, C., Goldenberg, D.L., Tugwell, P., Campbell, S.M., Abeles, M., Clark, P., Fam, A.G., Farber, S.J., Fiechtner, J.J., Franklin, C.M., Gatter, R.A., Hamaty, D., Lessard, J., Lichtbroun, A.S., Masi, A.T., McCain, G.A., Reynolds, W.J., Romano, T.J., Russell, I.J., & Sheon, R.P. (1990). The American College of Rheumatology 1990 criteria for the classification of fibromyalgia. *Arthritis and Rheumatism, 33*, 160-172.

Yeomans, J.D.I. & Conway, S.P. (1991). Biopsychosocial aspects of chronic fatigue syndrome (myalgic encephalomyelitis). *Journal of Infection, 23*, 263-269.

Depressive Comorbidity
in the Fatiguing Illnesses

Eleanor K. Axe, MD, PhD
Paul Satz, PhD

SUMMARY. Objective: The present study seeks to examine whether subjects with fatiguing illnesses and comorbid Major Depressive Disorder (MDD) have more symptoms than those without MDD.

Methods: The data was based on the Chronic Fatigue Syndrome (CFS) Surveillance System of the Centers for Disease Control and Prevention (CDC). Each of the 565 subjects enrolled in the study had a fatiguing illness and some had CFS. Subjects were evaluated for the duration and severity of the 11 symptoms and 3 physical signs listed in the 1988 CDC case definition (symptoms). They completed the Diagnostic Interview Schedule for the DSM-III-R which provided a diagnosis of several psychiatric disorders including MDD. Symptoms were compared in subjects with and without comorbid MDD.

Results: The mean number of symptoms was similar in the two groups. Three symptoms were found to be associated with MDD: neurobiological (cognitive complaints), sleep disturbance, and headache.

Eleanor K. Axe and Paul Satz are affiliated with the University of California, Los Angeles.

Address correspondence to: Eleanor K. Axe, MD, PhD, Arthur Ashe Student Health and Wellness Center, University of California, Los Angeles, Los Angeles, CA 90095.

The study utilizes the data set of the Chronic Fatigue Syndrome Surveillance System that was provided by James G. Dobbins, PhD of the Chronic Fatigue Syndrome Research Group, Division of Viral and Rickettsial Diseases, National Center for Infectious Diseases, Centers for Disease Control and Prevention, Atlanta, GA.

[Haworth co-indexing entry note]: "Depressive Comorbidity in the Fatiguing Illnesses." Axe, Eleanor K., and Paul Satz. Co-published simultaneously in *Journal of Chronic Fatigue Syndrome* (The Haworth Medical Press, an imprint of The Haworth Press, Inc.) Vol. 8, No. 3/4, 2001, pp. 23-29; and: *Innovations in Chronic Fatigue Syndrome Research and Clinical Practice* (ed: Roberto Patarca-Montero) The Haworth Medical Press, an imprint of The Haworth Press, Inc., 2001, pp. 23-29. Single or multiple copies of this article are available for a fee from The Haworth Document Delivery Service [1-800-342-9678, 9:00 a.m. - 5:00 p.m. (EST). E-mail address: getinfo@haworthpressinc. com].

Conclusions: Comorbid MDD in the fatiguing illnesses is not associated with a higher mean number of symptoms. In the present study a pattern of three individual symptoms emerged that was associated with comorbid MDD. It is suggested that subjects with fatiguing illnesses who have this symptom pattern be evaluated for comorbid MDD. *[Article copies available for a fee from The Haworth Document Delivery Service: 1-800-342-9678. E-mail address: <getinfo@haworthpressinc.com> Website: <http://www.HaworthPress.com> © 2001 by The Haworth Press, Inc. All rights reserved.]*

KEYWORDS. Depression, psychiatry, fatigue

INTRODUCTION

In the absence of an accepted biological marker for Chronic Fatigue Syndrome (CFS), case definitions were developed based on symptoms and physical signs. The 1988 CDC case definition includes 11 symptoms and 3 signs (1). The symptoms are: fever, sore throat, painful lymph nodes, muscle weakness, myalgia, post-exertional fatigue, headache, arthralgias, neurobiological (cognitive complaints), sleep disturbance, and sudden onset. The signs are: fever, pharyngitis, and palpable lymph nodes.

Concerns have been raised that the inclusion of a large number of symptoms in the case definition might result in a preferential selection of subjects with Major Depressive Disorder (MDD) into CFS studies (2-4). The present study seeks to examine whether subjects with fatiguing illnesses and comorbid MDD endorse more symptoms from the 1988 CDC case definition than those without comorbid depression.

METHOD

Participants

The present study uses the CFS Surveillance System of the CDC. This study followed an extremely careful subject selection process and generated extensive descriptive epidemiologic data on a large group of individuals according to strict eligibility criteria. The first entry criterion was debilitating fatigue (reduced activity, and greater effort required to accomplish one's usual activities). The second included two or more symptoms for six months (fever, sore throat, muscle weakness, unusual fatigue after exercise, tender lymph nodes, myalgia, and arthralgia) (5). These requirements were such that every subject in surveillance had a fatiguing illness.

The CDC enrolled 565 subjects from September 1989 to August 1993 at four geographic sites: Atlanta, Georgia; Wichita, Kansas; Grand Rapids, Michigan, and Reno, Nevada. The subjects were drawn from primary care settings. The demographic data suggest a mid-adult age at onset (Mean = 34; SD = 11.7). Subjects were mostly Caucasian (96.0%) and predominantly female (81.2%). Approximately 83% had an education beyond high school and 33.6% listed themselves as professional. The mean household income was $46,670 (SD = $28,832). The duration of illness suggested a chronic course (Mean = 6 years; SD = 7.34) (see Table 1).

Symptoms

The CDC did extensive interviews on each subject with respect to the symptoms listed in their 1988 case definition for CFS. In order for a symptom to be counted it had to meet criteria for duration, frequency, and severity (5).

Assessment Instruments

The CDC utilized a standardized psychosocial assessment instrument, the Diagnostic Interview Schedule (DIS) (6). It included questions that allowed for the diagnosis of several psychiatric disorders including Major Depressive Disorder. This structured interview was administered by nurses trained by CDC psychiatric personnel. A physician review committee confirmed the time of onset of the psychiatric disorders with medical records.

Subject Classification

The physician review committee classified its subjects into four diagnostic groups. Group I fully met the 1988 CDC case definition for CFS and included 130 subjects (23.0%). Group II had less fatigue severity, met fewer symptom criteria, and did not fully meet the case definition. It had 99 subjects (17.5%). In addition, the CDC project identified subjects with fatiguing illnesses where the committee felt that a different medical condition might have caused chronic fatigue and they were medically excluded from the 1988 case definition. Group III had 101 subjects (17.9%). Finally, Group IV included prior syndromal psychiatric disorders and consisted of 235 subjects (41.6%). When comparing diagnostic groups, Group II had milder symptoms, higher incomes, higher employment rates, and a higher proportion with children (see Table 1). These findings lend some credibility to the milder designation for Group II. Otherwise there were few differences across the diagnostic groups.

Analysis of Symptoms by MDD Status

Subjects were analyzed according to the mean number of symptoms adjusting for age, education, and gender, and compared by MDD status. Individual symptoms were studied to determine if a symptom pattern might be associated with MDD.

TABLE 1. Distribution of Population Characteristics by CDC Diagnostic Group[a]

	Group I (n = 130)		Group II (n = 99)		Group III (n = 101)		Group IV (n = 235)		Total (n = 565)		Analysis[b] F-value	p value
Mean Age at onset	30.42		32.00		37.75		35.26		34.02		9.90	0.0001
Mean duration-illness	5.29		7.51		5.49		6.90		6.00		0.52	0.6678
	No.	**%**	**No.**	**%**	**No.**	**%**	**No.**	**%**	**No.**	**%**	X^2	**p value**
Race/Ethnicity											0.509_{MH}[c]	0.476
Caucasian	124	96.9	96	98.0	91	92.9	220	96.1	531	96.0		
African American	2	1.6	1	1.0	2	2.0	3	1.3	8	1.5		
Latino	1	0.8	1	1.0	3	3.1	2	0.9	7	1.3		
Other	1	0.7	0	0.0	2	2.0	3	1.3	6	1.1		
Gender											3.432	0.330
Male	19	14.6	22	22.2	23	22.8	42	17.9	106	18.8		
Female	111	85.4	77	77.8	78	77.2	193	82.1	459	81.2		
Education											7.935	7.935
0-12 years	36	14.5	13	16.3	20	20.0	24	19.4	93	16.8		
13-15 years	104	41.8	39	48.8	50	50.0	49	39.5	242	43.8		
≥ 16 years	109	43.8	28	35.0	30	30.0	51	41.1	218	39.4		
Occupation											13.083	0.159
Professional	94	38.3	26	32.9	26	27.1	36	29.5	182	33.6		
Skill white collar	41	16.3	14	17.7	27	28.1	34	27.9	116	21.4		
Unskilled	90	36.7	33	41.7	38	39.6	46	37.7	207	38.2		
Other	20	8.1	6	7.5	5	5.2	6	4.9	37	6.8		
Income											34.085	0.001
$0-$20,000	21	8.9	22	29.3	23	25.0	30	26.6	96	18.4		
$20,001-$50,000	115	48.5	34	45.3	44	47.8	59	50.4	252	48.4		
≥ $50,001	101	42.6	19	25.3	25	27.2	28	23.9	173	33.2		

[a] Group I = CFS, Group II = mild, Group III = medical exclusion, Group IV = prior psychiatric disorder.
[b] The diagnostic groups differed by mean age at onset and mean age of subjects. They did not differ by mean duration of illness, race/ethnicity, gender or dominant hand.
[c] Mantel-Haenszel chi-square. Caucasians compared to *all* others.

RESULTS

Subjects with and without comorbid MDD endorsed a similar mean number of symptoms (T = +1.4, p = 0.2) after adjusting for age, education, and gender. Subjects with less education endorsed more symptoms (T = −2.3, p = 0.02). In the analysis of individual symptoms, a pattern emerged. Three symptoms were associated with MDD. They were: neurobiological (cognitive complaints) (OR = 3.5, CI = 1.6-7.6), sleep disturbance (OR = 1.7, CI = 1.1-2.7), and headache (OR = 1.4, CI = 1.0-2.0).

DISCUSSION

The present investigation was made possible because of the study's large sample size, the standardized testing instrument, and a careful categorization of subjects.

There were no differences in the adjusted mean numbers of symptoms in subjects with and without MDD. Since subjects with less education had more symptoms, it is recommended that educational levels be taken into account when symptoms are evaluated. With respect to individual symptom patterns, the association of MDD with neurobehavioral (cognitive complaints), sleep disorders, headache suggests that if subjects endorse this symptom pattern that they be evaluated for MDD. In an earlier study (7) the symptom pattern associated with MDD differed from the pattern associated with cognitive impairment. Subjects with these two symptom patterns differed in functional disability as measured by Sickness Impact Profile test scores. In that study cognitive complaints were not found to be associated with cognitive impairment. Our findings warrant a more systematic replication to clarify the role of the individual symptoms in the fatiguing illnesses.

It is suggested that future studies compare CFS and non-CFS subjects by MDD status and cognitive functioning using brain imaging, immunologic, histopathologic, and other biological surveys. Such studies may further clarify the roles of MDD and cognitive functioning in CFS.

While this study provides some new insights into the MDD correlates of CFS, there are concerns that could limit some of the conclusions.

First, this study was administratively based. It included subjects seeking care, who agreed to participate, and were selected by physicians who believed that CFS was a diagnosable disorder (8,9). Compared to population-based prevalence studies (10-13) these subjects were largely Caucasian. Our findings should be restricted to Caucasians. Second, this study reported prevalence cases. Due to the chronic nature of CFS, prevalence is a more convenient measure than incidence. However, it is not the most desirable measure. Associations found using prevalence measures may not reflect determinants related to etiology but rather consequences of illness (14). Incidence data should provide more accurate estimates of the relationship of MDD to CFS (15). Finally, the present study did not compare the DIS to other structured clinical interviews. It is not known which structured clinical interview instrument might provide the most accurate assessment of psychiatric disorders in CFS (3). Each of these problems in subject selection or measurement could reduce the interpretability of the findings.

REFERENCES

1. Holmes GP, Kaplan JE, Gantz NM, Komaroff AL, Schonberger LB, Straus SE, Jones, JF, Dubois RE, Cunningham-Rundles C, Pahwa, Tostato G, Zegans LS, Purtilo DT, Brown N, Schooley RT, Brus, I. Chronic fatigue syndrome: a working case definition. Ann Intern Med 1988; 108: 387-9.

2. Katon W, Russo J. Chronic fatigue syndrome criteria. A critique of the requirement for multiple physical complaints.

3. Jason LA, King CP, Richman JA, Taylor RR, Torres SR, Song S. US case definition of chronic fatigue syndrome: diagnostic and theoretical issues. J Chronic Fatigue Syndrome 1999; 5 (3-4): 3-33.

4. Lloyd A. Chronic fatigue and chronic fatigue syndrome: shifting boundaries and attributions. Amer J Med 1998; 105 (3A): 7-10S.

5. Reyes M, Gary HE, Dobbins JG, Randall B, Steele L, Fukuda K, et al. Surveillance for chronic fatigue syndrome-four U.S. cities, September 1989 through August 1993. Morbid Mortal Wkly Rep, CDC Surveillance Summaries, 1997;46 Suppl 1. (SS-2): 3-14.

6. Robins LN, Helzer MD, Croughan J, Ratcliff KS. National Institute of Mental Health Diagnostic Interview Schedule: its history, characteristics and validity. Arch Gen Psychiatry 1981; 38: 381-9.

7. Axe E. Neuropsychological and Psychiatric Correlates in Chronic Fatigue Syndrome [dissertation]. Los Angeles (CA): University of California at Los Angeles; 1999.

8. Gunn W, Connell D, Randall DB. Epidemiology of chronic fatigue syndrome: the Centers for Disease Control Study. In: Bock G, Whelan J, editors. Chronic fatigue syndrome Ciba Foundation Symposium, 173, Chichester: John Wiley and Sons; 1993. pp. 83-101.

9. Reyes M. An epidemiologic investigation of chronic fatigue syndrome [dissertation]. Berkeley (CA): Univ. of California at Berkeley; 1995.

10. Buchwald D, Umali P, Umali J, Kith P, Pearlman T, Komaroff AL. Chronic fatigue and the chronic fatigue syndrome: prevalence in a Pacific northwest health care system. Ann Intern Med 1995; 123 (2): 81-8.

11. Jason LA, Taylor R, Wagner L, Holden J, Ferrari JR. Estimating rates of chronic fatigue syndrome from a community-based sample: a pilot study. Am J Community Psychol 1995; 23: 557-68.

12. Shefer A, Dobbins JG, Fukuda K, Steele L, Koo D, Nisenbaum R, Rutherford G. Fatiguing illness among employees in three large state office buildings, California, 1993: was there an outbreak? J Psychiatric Res 1997; 31 (1): 31-43.

13. Steele L, Dobbins JG, Fukuda K, Reyes M, Randall B, Koppleman M, Reeves WC. The epidemiology of chronic fatigue in San Francisco. Am J Med 1998; 105 (3A): 83-90S.

14. Rothman KJ, Greenland S. Modern Epidemiology. 2nd ed. Philadelphia (PA): Lippencott-Raven; 1998. pp. 44-5.

15. Reyes M, Nisenbaum R, Stewart G, Reeves WC. Update: Wichita population-based study of fatiguing illness. Proceedings of the Symposium: Fourth International Research, Clinical and Patient Conference, American Association for Chronic Fatigue Syndrome; 1998 Oct. 10-12; Cambridge, Massachusetts.

Measuring Attributions
About Chronic Fatigue Syndrome

Leonard A. Jason, PhD
Renée R. Taylor, PhD

SUMMARY. Three studies explored the effects of different diagnostic labels and different types of recommended treatments for Chronic Fatigue Syndrome upon attributions regarding its cause, nature, severity, contagion, prognosis, and treatment. Attributions for Chronic Fatigue Syndrome appear to change based upon the diagnostic label given for the syndrome and the type of treatment recommended. Results suggest that, in comparison to the Chronic Fatigue Syndrome label, the Myalgic Encephalopathy label prompts attributions that this syndrome is a serious condition associated with a physiologically-based etiology, a poor prognosis, and decreased potential for organ donation. Results also suggest that, compared with cognitive coping skills treatment, treatment with ampligen appears to be associated with perceptions of Chronic Fatigue Syndrome as an accurate diagnosis and as a severely disabling condition. *[Article copies available for a fee from The Haworth Document Delivery Service: 1-800-342-9678. E-mail address: <getinfo@haworthpressinc.com> Website: <http://www.HaworthPress.com> © 2001 by The Haworth Press, Inc. All rights reserved.]*

KEYWORDS. Attributions, Ampligen, Myalgic Encephalomyelitis

Leonard A. Jason and Renée R. Taylor are affiliated with the Department of Psychology, DePaul University.

Financial support for this study was provided by NIAID grant number AI36295.

Address correspondence to: Leonard A. Jason, PhD, Department of Psychology, DePaul University, 2219 North Kenmore, Chicago, IL 60614.

[Haworth co-indexing entry note]: "Measuring Attributions About Chronic Fatigue Syndrome." Jason, Lenoard A., and Renée R. Taylor. Co-published simultaneously in *Journal of Chronic Fatigue Syndrome* (The Haworth Medical Press, an imprint of The Haworth Press, Inc.) Vol. 8, No. 3/4, 2001, pp. 31-40; and: *Innovations in Chronic Fatigue Syndrome Research and Clinical Practice* (ed: Roberto Patarca-Montero) The Haworth Medical Press, an imprint of The Haworth Press, Inc., 2001, pp. 31-40. Single or multiple copies of this article are available for a fee from The Haworth Document Delivery Service [1-800-342-9678, 9:00 a.m. - 5:00 p.m. (EST). E-mail address: getinfo@haworthpressinc.com].

The presence of stigma among individuals with Chronic Fatigue Syndrome (CFS) has been formally assessed by several investigators. For example, Green, Romei, and Natelson (1999) found that 95% of individuals seeking medical treatment for CFS reported feelings of estrangement, 70% believed that others attributed their CFS symptoms to psychological causes, 39% felt a need to be secretive about their symptoms in certain circumstances, and many participants reported having been labeled as having a primary psychological difficulty by one or more physicians consulted. Anderson and Ferrans (1997) found that 77% of individuals with CFS reported past negative experiences with health care providers. Survey findings from a CFS organization indicated that 57% of respondents were treated badly or very badly by their doctors (David, Wessely, and Pelosi, 1991).

There is a relationship between beliefs about the degree to which people with CFS are responsible for their illness, beliefs about the relevance of CFS as a valid illness, and beliefs about the personality traits of people with CFS. For example, Shlaes, Jason and Ferrari (1999) found that if someone believes that people with CFS are responsible for their illness, it is likely that they will also believe that people with CFS have negative personality characteristics, such as being compulsive or overly driven. It is possible that negative attitudes might be a function of past government and media portrayals of CFS as either non-existent or as a function of a neurotic, overworked, stressed lifestyle, as was depicted in the labels such as the "Yuppie Flu" (Jason et al., 1997). It is also possible that the negative stigma that is associated with CFS could in part be due to the trivializing name that has been given to this disorder. The name selected to characterize an illness, such as Chronic Fatigue Syndrome, can influence how patients are perceived and ultimately treated by medical personnel, family members and work associates.

The patient community has felt that the term Chronic Fatigue Syndrome trivializes the seriousness of this illness, as the illness is typified by many severe symptoms in addition to fatigue, and fatigue is generally regarded as a common symptom experienced by many otherwise healthy individuals in the general population (Taylor, Friedberg, & Jason, 2001). In addition, CFS is frequently confused with chronic fatigue, which is a symptom of many illnesses, including some psychiatric disorders. Although it was expected that the CFS name would be eventually replaced as more information became available, this name has remained and has become the most commonly used label within the United States (Friedberg & Jason, 1998).

During the summer of 1997, The Chronic Fatigue and Immune Dysfunction Syndrome (CFIDS) Association of America conducted a survey of its members to determine their opinion about changing the name CFS. Eighty-five percent of respondents indicated they wanted the name changed (Name-Change Survey Results, 1997). Another survey of 182 respondents by the editor of a newsletter indicated that 92% wanted the CFS name changed (Burns, 1998). Many medical personnel and research scientists feel that if the name were to be changed, it would be best to have a scientific basis for the change. Unfortunately, few data have been collected to help guide the process of revising the name.

Two studies reviewed herein investigated whether different names for CFS indeed prompt different attributions regarding its cause, nature, severity, contagion, prognosis, and recommended treatment among samples of medical trainees and university undergraduates.

STUDIES 1 AND 2

During the Fall of 1998 and the Winter and Spring of 1999, 105 medical trainees were randomly assigned to one of three conditions, each prompting them with one of three different diagnostic labels for CFS (Jason, Taylor, Plioplys, Stepanek, Shlaes, in press). The same case study of a patient with prototypical symptoms of CFS was presented to all participants across the three name conditions. The only difference between the three conditions involved the name given for the illness described in the case study. For one third of the trainees, the patient was labeled as having CFS. For another third of the trainees, the patient was labeled as having Florence Nightingale Disease (FN), and for the final third of the trainees, the patient was labeled as having Myalgic Encephalopathy (ME). The current label, CFS, was originally given to define a poorly understood pattern of symptoms forming a syndrome characterized by prominent fatigue. The second label, Florence Nightingale Disease, is an eponym, a name given to characterize an illness by associating it with a well-known person who either had the illness or discovered it. One example of a commonly used eponym is Lou Gehrig's Disease (ALS). Florence Nightingale Disease has been used as an eponym for CFS, since Florence Nightingale, a nurse well known for improving public health during the Crimean War, became very ill following the war and spent the remainder of her life confined to bed and sofa due to chronic fatigue. The third label, Myalgic Encephalopathy, is a medically-based term commonly used to characterize CFS in the United

Kingdom, and proposed for use in the United States by various patient groups.

During the Winter and Spring of 1999, 141 female and male undergraduates of diverse academic backgrounds taking an introduction to psychology course at a large university in Chicago participated in the same study (Jason, Taylor, Stepanek, & Plioplys, in press). Each undergraduate was randomly assigned to one of the three conditions. As in the medical trainee sample, the identical case study describing a patient with classic symptoms of CFS was presented across the three name conditions: CFS, Florence Nightingale Disease, and Myalgic Encephalopathy.

After reading the case study, participants in both the medical trainee and undergraduate samples responded to a written series of questions examining the causality, diagnosis, severity, contagion, prognosis, and treatment of the patient's illness.

RESULTS

For the question, "What is the likelihood that the person is correctly diagnosed," there was a significant difference between the three groups [X^2 (2, $N = 105$) = 10.48, $p < 0.01$]. Fifty-four percent of individuals in the CFS condition indicated that the person was likely or very likely to have been correctly diagnosed, as compared with 28% and 19% from the ME and FN conditions, respectively. There were also significant differences among the three name conditions for the question assessing the likelihood that this illness was the result of an undiscovered infection, cancer or other illness [X^2 (2, $N = 105$) = 5.84, $p < 0.05$]. Forty-seven percent of those in the FN condition indicated that it was likely or very likely that the illness was the result of an undiscovered infection, cancer, or other illness, whereas only 28% and 22% of those in the ME and CFS responded in this way. Lastly, for the question assessing the likelihood that the patient will improve within the next two years, there was a significant difference between the three name conditions [X^2 (2, $N = 105$) = 6.51, $p < 0.05$]. Forty-two percent and 41% responded that it was likely or very likely that the patient would improve in the FN and CFS conditions, respectively, but only 16% in the ME condition thought it was likely or very likely that the patient would improve.

When we added the undergraduate sample to these analyses, similar findings as above occurred in terms of diagnostic accuracy and considering the patient as a candidate for organ donation. In addition, compared with the CFS name condition, the ME name condition predicted more medical (physiological) attributions for the illness than psychiatric explanations. A significantly higher proportion of medical trainees in comparison to the undergraduates were likely to characterize the illness as primary depression (72.4% versus 27.6%) and were likely to think that the patient would attempt suicide (83.8% versus 16.2%).

The undergraduates viewed the patient's cognitive impairment as significantly more severe that did the medical trainees, were significantly less likely to consider the patient as a candidate for organ donation, were significantly more likely to believe that precautions should be taken to avoid contagion, and were significantly more likely to think that the patient was malingering than the medical trainees. The medical trainees rated the patient's quality of life as significantly poorer than the undergraduates. Finally, the medical trainee group was significantly more likely to have heard of CFS than the undergraduate group. Ninety-three percent of the medical trainees heard of CFS, as compared with 65.0% of the undergraduates.

STUDY 3

Ninety-three practicing mental health practitioners (social work interns, clinical psychology externs, interns, and post-doctoral fellows, licensed clinical social workers, and licensed clinical psychologists) were recruited for participation from three Chicago-area outpatient mental health centers that serve as training sites for mental health professionals (91.4% of the sample) and from two psychological conferences (8.6% of the sample) (Taylor, Jason, Kennedy & Friedberg, in press).

Participants were randomly assigned to one of three conditions, each reflecting one of three different types of currently recommended treatment for CFS. With the exception of manipulation in type of treatment recommended, the identical case study of a woman with prototypic CFS symptoms (i.e., low-grade fever, headaches, sore throat, muscle and joint pains, tender and swollen lymph nodes, and a constant feeling of fatigue) diagnosed with CFS by a physician, was given to all participants to read across conditions.

The description of *Ampligen* treatment explained that it was an experimental drug (an immune system modulator) expected to improve functioning and decrease symptoms in severely disabled patients with sudden onset of symptoms and cognitive deficits. The drug was administered intravenously, with possible side effects during the first three months, including an increase in headaches, nausea, and/or pain.

The *Cognitive-Behavioral Therapy with Graded Activity* treatment explained that its objective was to have the patient view her illness as non-organic in origin, with a focus on increasing, rather than avoiding activity. Cognitive-behavioral therapy is based on the hypothesis that inaccurate beliefs, ineffective coping behaviors, negative moods, social problems, and pathophysiological processes interact to perpetuate the illness. The patient in this condition was encouraged to question the explanation that her illness was caused by a virus, to consider psychological and social factors as reasonable alternative explanations, and utilize more effective coping strategies to improve daily functioning.

The *Cognitive Coping Skills Therapy* (Friedberg, 1995) treatment focussed on the identification of symptom relapse triggers, activity moderation to minimize setbacks, acquisition of cognitive and behavioral coping skills, stress reduction, and social support. This treatment was intended to help the patient learn to manage her symptoms, since an effective biomedical intervention had not been discovered. The description also stated that this therapy may indirectly effect immune system functioning via stress reduction.

All participants were asked to complete a brief questionnaire assessing their attributions about the etiology, diagnostic accuracy, severity, contagion, prognosis, and expected treatment outcome regarding the woman's illness.

RESULTS

Participants in the Ampligen condition were significantly more likely to think that the patient was correctly diagnosed as having CFS [F (2, 92) = 3.18, $p < .05$] and also thought the patient was significantly more disabled than did individuals in the Cognitive-Behavioral Therapy with Graded Activity condition [F (2, 92) = 3.20, $p < .05$].

DISCUSSION

In the first two studies, three different diagnostic labels (Chronic Fatigue Syndrome, Florence Nightingale Disease, and Myalgic Encephalopathy) were tested to determine their effects upon the attributions of medical trainees and college undergraduates regarding Chronic Fatigue Syndrome. Participants were divided into three groups, with the only difference between groups being in the type of diagnostic label given as the diagnosis for a patient described in a case study read by all participants. Results of the first two studies suggested that participant's attributions about CFS change based upon the different diagnostic labels used to characterize it. While medical trainees viewed the Chronic Fatigue Syndrome label as the most accurate diagnosis based on the case history described, the Myalgic Encephalopathy label was associated with the poorest prognosis. When undergraduates were added to the analysis, those prompted with the Myalgic Encephalopathy label were more likely to attribute a physiological cause to the illness, and less likely to consider the patient in the case study as a potential candidate for organ donation than those prompted with the Chronic Fatigue Syndrome label.

The CFS name was predictably considered the term that represented the most accurate diagnosis. This finding may, in part, be explained by the fact that, in contrast to the labels of Florence Nightingale Disease or Myalgic Encephalopathy, the CFS label is most commonly used in both medical and lay communities within the United States.

In addition to issues surrounding the accuracy of the name given for the syndrome, findings indicated that individuals appear to differ in their attributions about certain aspects of the illness depending upon their educational context (medical training versus multidisciplinary undergraduate training) and, potentially, depending upon their familiarity with CFS. In general, findings indicated that, in contrast to the undergraduates, the medical trainees (advanced medical students and residents) were more familiar with CFS and were significantly more likely than the undergraduates to associate the illness with poorer quality of life, regardless of whether it was labeled CFS, Florence Nightingale Disease, or Myalgic Encephalopathy. In addition, the medical trainees were significantly less likely to view the prototypic patient as malingering when compared with the undergraduates. These findings may be due to increased training and experience in treating and learning about the complexities of various symptom patterns and illnesses among medical trainees.

Contrary to these findings and explanations, however, the medical trainees were significantly less likely to believe that precautions should be taken to avoid contagion as compared with the undergraduates. Furthermore, the medical trainees were significantly more likely to consider the patient as a candidate for organ donation. Taken together, these findings may, in part, be attributable to increased knowledge about issues related to contagion and organ donation among the medical trainees. Since there were no objective laboratory findings, the medical trainees may have considered contagion as less of a risk factor. These results may also reflect a decreased tendency to believe in an underlying physiological cause and organ-related pathology among the medical trainees.

Findings indicating that the medical trainees were significantly more likely than the undergraduates to think that the prototypic patient was suffering from primary depression, rather than being physically ill, support the suggestion that medical professionals in training may be less likely to believe in the physiological nature of the illness. The medical trainees were also significantly more likely to think that the patient would attempt suicide than the undergraduates.

Other findings suggest that medical trainees in particular are significantly more likely to characterize CFS as primary depression than undergraduates, and, possibly as a result, are significantly more likely to associate the illness with suicide attempt. Further research is clearly needed to test potential explanations for these findings, and to determine whether they would replicate for more experienced medical professionals no longer receiving formal training.

Given previous findings for feelings of stigmatization among individuals with CFS and frequent perceptions that medical professionals either minimize the severity of CFS, or attribute it to psychological factors (Romei et al., 1996), some of the findings presented herein are optimistic in that they indicate that medical professionals in training are significantly less likely than undergraduates to consider CFS patients to be malingering, and are significantly more willing to view individuals with the illness as having a poorer quality of life.

Results of the third investigation support the hypothesis that physician recommendation for treatment of CFS can influence subsequent attributions about the illness among mental health practitioners. When a medically-based treatment (Ampligen) was recommended, the practitioners were significantly more likely to believe that the patient was correctly diagnosed with Chronic Fatigue Syndrome and significantly more disabled than those prompted with recommendation for a psychologically-based treatment (Cognitive-Behavior Therapy with Graded Activity). These findings highlight distinctions in attributions that can result from recommending a medically-based orientation toward CFS treatment, versus one based heavily on minimizing medical factors, emphasizing psychiatric factors, and increasing activity levels.

Physicians who recommend psychotherapy in the absence of other medical recommendations may be unwittingly contributing to a resulting over-emphasis on psychiatric interpretations and minimization of symptom severity and disability by mental health practitioners working with these patients, particularly when the form of psychotherapy recommended involves discounting medical explanations. Prior research involving people with AIDS has demonstrated the importance of the role of empathy in improving attitudes toward members of stigmatized groups (Batson et al., 1997). Since mental health providers typically provide cognitive behavioral therapy and other forms of psychotherapy to patients, future research and practice should focus upon educating mental health trainees and clinicians working in rehabilitation-oriented settings about the complex nature of chronic fatigue syndrome, and about the importance of maintaining a balanced understanding of the illness and of the range of possible treatment options. Given that ambiguity about the nature of a given condition can lead to misattributions, another important clinical implication of the findings is that, when dealing with a relatively new clinical entity such as CFS, it is important for mental health professionals to work in closer collaboration with physicians to assure clearest communication of symptoms, rationale for treatment, and any complicating factors unique to the patient in question.

These preliminary studies represent the first efforts of their kind to test the impact of diagnostic labels and physician treatment recommendations upon attributions made by undergraduates and health care providers. These studies can serve as a paradigm for future research into the roles of covert stigma, diagnostic labeling, physician diagnosis, and treatment recommendations in the conduct of research, treatment and psychotherapy by health care providers. Future research is necessary to demonstrate the role of attributions about CFS in influencing the strength of the patient-provider relationship, and the overall effectiveness of various forms of rehabilitative intervention with this illness population.

REFERENCES

Anderson, J.S. & Ferrans, C.E. (1997). The quality of life of persons with chronic fatigue syndrome. *Journal of Nervous and Mental Disease, 185,* 359-367.

Batson, C.D., Polycarpou, M.P., Harmon-Jones, E., Imhoff, H.J., Mitchener, E.C., Bednar, L.L., Klein, T.R., & Highberger, L. (1997). Empathy and attitudes: Can feeling for a member of a stigmatized group improve feelings toward the group? *Journal of Personality and Social Psychology, 72,* 105-118.

David, A.S., Wessely, S., & Pelosi, A.J. (1991). Chronic fatigue syndrome: Signs of a new approach. *British Journal of Hospital Medicine, 45,* 158-163.

Friedberg, F., & Jason, L.A. (1998). *Understanding chronic fatigue syndrome: An empirical guide to assessment and treatment.* Washington, D.C.: American Psychological Association.

Friedberg, F. (1996). Chronic Fatigue Syndrome: A new clinical application. *Professional Psychology: Research and Practice, 27,* 487-494.

Green, J., Romei, J., & Natelson, B.J. (1999). Stigma and chronic fatigue syndrome. *Journal of Chronic Fatigue Syndrome, 5,* 63-75.

Jason, L.A., Richman, J.A., Friedberg, F., Wagner, L., Taylor, R., & Jordan, K.M. (1997). Politics, science, and the emergence of a new disease: The case of Chronic Fatigue Syndrome. *American Psychologist, 52,* 973-983.

Jason, L.A., Taylor, R.R., Plioplys, S., Stepanek, Z., & Shlaes, J. (in press). Evaluating attributions for an illness based upon the name: Chronic Fatigue Syndrome, Myalgic Encephalopathy and Florence Nightingale Disease. *American Journal of Community Psychology.*

Jason, L.A., Taylor, R.R., Stepanek, Z., & Plioplys, S. (in press). Attitudes regarding chronic fatigue syndrome: The importance of a name. *Journal of Health Psychology.*

Name-Change Survey Results (1997). http://www.cfids.org/chronicle/97summer/survey.html

Romei, J., Green, J., & Heinzen, T. (1996). *Perceived stigma in chromic fatigue syndrome.* Paper presented at the 1996 Meeting of the Eastern Psychological Association, Philadelphia, PA.

Shlaes, J.L., Jason, L.A., & Ferrari, J. (1999). The development of the Chronic Fatigue Syndrome Attitudes Test: A psychometric analysis. *Evaluation and the Health Professions, 22,* 442-465.

Taylor, R.R., Friedberg, F., & Jason, L.A. (in press). *A clinician's guide to controversial illnesses: Chronic fatigue syndrome, Fibromyalgia, and Multiple Chemical Sensitivities.* Sarasota, FL: Professional Resource Press.

Taylor, R.R., Jason, L.A., Kennedy, C.L., & Friedberg, F. (in press). Evaluating attributions for chronic fatigue syndrome based upon type of treatment recommended. *Rehabilitation Psychology.*

Health-Related Personality Variables in Chronic Fatigue Syndrome and Multiple Sclerosis

Susan K. Johnson, PhD
Gudrun Lange, PhD
Lana Tiersky, PhD
John DeLuca, PhD
Benjamin H. Natelson, MD

SUMMARY. This study investigated personality variables in patients with Chronic Fatigue Syndrome (CFS) and Multiple Sclerosis (MS), with healthy, sedentary subjects as controls. CFS and MS groups were higher on alexithymia, characterized as difficulty in describing and differentiating emotions and marked externalization. CFS and MS groups reported a more depressive attributional style than healthy participants, reflecting beliefs that causes for good events are not diffused into other areas of life while causes for bad events will always be present. The CFS group was significantly lower on doctors/others locus of control indicating lack of trust in medical professionals. Results indicate that CFS and

---

Susan K. Johnson is affiliated with the University of North Carolina-Charlotte.

Gudrun Lange, John DeLuca, and Benjamin H. Natelson are affiliated with the University of Medicine & Dentistry of New Jersey.

Lana Tiersky is affiliated with the Department of Psychology, Fairleigh Dickinson University, Teaneck, NJ 07666.

This study was supported in part by the Pilot Project program of the CFS Cooperative Research Center (NIH U01AI-32247).

[Haworth co-indexing entry note]: "Health-Related Personality Variables in Chronic Fatigue Syndrome and Multiple Sclerosis." Johnson, Susan K. et al. Co-published simultaneously in *Journal of Chronic Fatigue Syndrome* (The Haworth Medical Press, an imprint of The Haworth Press, Inc.) Vol. 8, No. 3/4, 2001, pp. 41-52; and: *Innovations in Chronic Fatigue Syndrome Research and Clinical Practice* (ed: Roberto Patarca-Montero) The Haworth Medical Press, an imprint of The Haworth Press, Inc., 2001, pp. 41-52. Single or multiple copies of this article are available for a fee from The Haworth Document Delivery Service [1-800-342-9678, 9:00 a.m. - 5:00 p.m. (EST). E-mail address: getinfo@haworthpressinc.com].

MS are similar to each other while different from the healthy group on certain personality variables that likely reflect the demoralizing effects of coping with a chronic, disabling illness marked by uncertainty. *[Article copies available for a fee from The Haworth Document Delivery Service: 1-800-342-9678. E-mail address: <getinfo@haworthpressinc.com> Website: <http://www. HaworthPress.com> © 2001 by The Haworth Press, Inc. All rights reserved.]*

KEYWORDS. Chronic Fatigue Syndrome, Multiple Sclerosis, alexithymia, locus of control, attributional style, hardiness

INTRODUCTION

The focus of the present study was to compare personality variables that relate to health in patients with Chronic Fatigue Syndrome (CFS) and Multiple Sclerosis as well as healthy controls. CFS and MS share a number of symptoms such as fatigue, depression, and neuropsychological difficulties yet the etiology of CFS is unresolved whereas etiology in MS is known to be neuropathologic.

Previous studies of psychological factors in CFS have focused on DSM III-R symptom (Axis I) disorders and found relatively high rates in CFS subjects (1-3) whereas fewer studies have examined personality variables in this population. Studies of personality in chronic fatigue (CF) populations have shown a tendency for histrionic and emotional traits to be overrepresented in chronic fatigue subjects. Yet, these studies suffered methodological flaws ranging from lack of a control group (4) using the MMPI without correcting for physical symptoms (5,6) and not using CDC criteria CFS subjects. Pepper et al. (7) examined Axis I and Axis II disorders in subjects with chronic fatigue, MS and major depression. They reported that the CF group had significantly less depression and fewer personality disorders than the depressed group. The CF and MS groups did not differ in the rate of personality disorders, although the CF group had significantly more frequent current depression than the MS group. Johnson et al. (8) similarly examined Axis I and II disorders, used assessment instruments not contaminated by physical symptom items, included only CDC criteria CFS subjects, and also examined trait neuroticism. Subjectively reported symptoms have been shown to be systematically biased by neuroticism, which is strongly correlated with health complaints but not actual health status (9). The depressed group was found to have significantly more personality disorders and elevated neuroticism scores compared with the CFS, MS, and healthy groups. The CFS and MS subjects had intermediary scores, which were significantly higher than the healthy controls (8).

In addition to Axis I and II pathology, individual differences along personality variables other than neuroticism may be important in understanding CFS. For instance, CFS patients may display a personality style that renders them more vulnerable to stresses of daily life, which consequently enhances their susceptibility to chronic illness. Numerous studies have found a positive relationship between stress, depression, and altered immune function in other fatiguing illnesses, including Rheumatoid Arthritis (10), Multiple Sclerosis (11), and Lupus (12). Thus, in the present study we assessed appraisal of current stress.

The personality variables of hardiness, perceived locus of control, and attributional style have been shown to influence health and chronic illness. Hardiness is a personality style thought to moderate stress-illness relationships; it consists of three components: commitment (vs. alienation), control (vs. powerlessness), and challenge (vs. threat). The hardy individual is expected to perceive situational stress in a positive and active manner, thereby reducing psychological strain and promoting mental and physical health (13). The measure of locus of control (LOC) assesses whether an individual perceives control over life events (14), i.e., chronic illness, to be determined by internal or external forces. Externally oriented patients tend to be more physically symptomatic and engage in more health-seeking behavior (5,15). An outward style of attribution is associated with helplessness, increased fatigue, lack of self-efficacy, and diminished responsibility for one's own health. We specifically measured health locus of control (16) which measures chance, internality as well as a doctors/others component.

Although depression has been suggested as an explanation for CFS, studies in our lab have found CFS and MS participants differ from clinically depressed participants on the Beck Depression Inventory. The Beck Depression Inventory (BDI) was used to determine the extent and pattern of depressive symptomatology among participants with CFS, MS and depression (17) employing the method of Huber et al. (18) which divides the BDI into four categories, mood, self-reproach, somatic, and vegetative symptoms to compare these specific characteristics of depression. Analysis of symptoms as a percentage of total BDI revealed no significant differences in mood or vegetative items. However, the CFS and MS groups exhibited a significantly lower percentage of self-reproach symptoms than DEP, whereas the DEP group showed a lower percentage of somatic symptoms than the CFS and MS groups. A depressive cognitive style of learned helplessness has been found to be related to poor health outcomes (19). Thus, in the present study we examined whether individuals with CFS or MS displayed learned helplessness wherein an individual makes stable, global and personal attributions for events.

Alexithymia is a personality construct that may have some relevance for CFS. Alexithymia is a multidimensional construct that includes lack of awareness of emotions, difficulty distinguishing emotions from bodily sensations, difficulty verbalizing emotions, and marked externalization (20). This difficulty in expressing and discriminating emotions could lead to misinterpreting emotional distress as physical distress in CFS symptom reporting. Clinical observations of over 100 CFS patients in the UK revealed a typical premorbid characterization of an individual who along with high achievement standards and perfectionistic tendencies, also tends to "bottle up feelings" (21).

The following study attempted to clarify whether the health-related personality variables of perceived stress, hardiness, locus of control, attributional style or alexithymia would differentiate individuals with CFS from either another chronic illness group (MS) or healthy controls. A tenacity in organic illness conviction among individuals with CFS has been noted by several investigators (22,23), so additionally, attributions for CFS have been characterized for this sample.

METHOD

Subjects

CFS (N = 22), MS (N = 16), and healthy, sedentary subjects (N = 16) for this study were recruited through participants enrolled in ongoing research studies at the New Jersey Chronic Fatigue Syndrome Center. Participants who had been examined at the Center within the past 6 months were contacted. Demographic characteristics are presented in Table 1, the MS subjects were significantly older $F(2, 53) = 4.1$, p = 0.02, there were no differences in level of education ($F(2, 53) = 2.3$; p = .08) or in gender distribution (Fisher's exact test, p = .89) (Table 1). Healthy subjects were recruited from advertisements in the community. MS subjects were referred from the MS clinic at UMDNJ-New Jersey Medical School and were classified with clinically definite MS (24). The mean EDSS score for the MS group was 4.5 (SEM = 0.57), indicating a moderate level of disability. MS subjects had a significantly

TABLE 1. Demographic Data (Mean ± SEM)

	M	N F	Age	Range	Education	Range
CFS	2	20	38.5 ± 2.2	18-53 yrs	15.6 ± 0.6	9-20
MS	5	11	48.6 ± 3.5*	23-68 yrs	15.4 ± 0.6	12-19
HEA	3	13	39.7 ± 2.1	25-54 yrs	14.6 ± 0.4	12-18

greater disease duration (11.5 ± 3.3 years) than CFS subjects ($4.13 \pm .43$ years), t $(1,36) = 2.6$, p $= .01$.

CFS patients were either self or physician referred to the CFS Center at UMDNJ. Potential CFS subjects were accepted as research participants following a careful history, physical examination, and elimination of possible medical causes of fatigue (25,26). CFS subjects were not paid, but they received their medical work up for free as compensation for their participation. To be accepted as subjects, CFS patients had to report sustained fatigue severe enough to have reduced activity by at least 50%, lasting at least 6 months and not explained by other known medical causes. Also, patients had to endorse at least 8 of the 11 minor symptoms and signs whose presence are required as part of the CDC case definition for CFS. To count toward diagnosis, these symptoms had to have produced a significant problem in the patient's life in the month prior to their visit.

Procedure

The recruitment procedure consisted of sending introductory letters describing the study to chronic fatigue syndrome, multiple sclerosis patients, and healthy, sedentary controls recently enrolled in the NJ CFS Center. All potential subjects contacted in this way were asked to indicate on a postcard whether they prefer *not* to participate in the study. Those patients who did not decline participation in the study were sent: (1) a cover letter further explaining the study and a number to call with any questions they might have about the study; (2) a set of questionnaires; and (3) two copies of the Informed Consent, one to sign and return with the completed questionnaires in a postage paid return envelope should the subjects wish to participate, and one to keep. A total of 43 questionnaire packets were sent to individuals with CFS and 24 were returned (56% response rate). Twenty-six were sent to healthy subjects and 16 were returned (61% response rate), while 16 of the 18 packets were sent to individuals with MS were returned (88% response rate). There were no differences between the CFS participants who returned questionnaires on age $t(1, 39) = 0.43$, $p = 0.66$, education $t(1, 38) = 0.04$, $p = 0.96$, or gender distribution, nor were there any differences in the healthy participants who returned questionnaires on age $t(1, 24) = 0.57$, $p = 0.58$, education $t(1, 24) = 0.36$, $p = 0.71$ or gender distribution.

Questionnaires:

1. Perceived Stress Scale (PSS)–This is a 14 item scale designed to measure the degree to which situations in one's own life are appraised as stressful. The PSS has been shown to be reliable, and to measure a construct independent of depression (27). The scale yields a single score and a higher score is indicative of greater levels of perceived stress.
2. Personal Views Survey–This 50-item hardiness measure yields a composite hardiness score, as well as scores on the three components of commitment, control, and challenge (28).
3. Health Locus of Control (Form C)–This locus of control measure contains 18 items made up of belief statements concerning health. There are three subscales that ascribe control to internal forces, the external forces of chance, or doctors and other people (16). The score on each subscale is the sum of the values circled for each item on the subscale.
4. Attributional Style Questionnaire (ASQ)–This 48-item scale is used in determining the degree to which the subject attributes positive and negative situations to internal, stable, and global forces. The ASQ presents subjects with six bad events (e.g., you meet a friend who acts hostilely toward you; you can't get all the work done that others expect of you) and six good events (e.g., you do a project that is highly praised; you meet a friend who compliments you on your appearance). Participants rate the cause of each event on a 7-point scale according to its internality versus externality, stability versus instability, and globality versus specificity. Situations are interpersonal or achievement related (29).
5. Toronto Alexithymia Scale–This is a 26-item scale which yields a composite score on the degree to which subjects are able to discriminate between emotional and physical distress (30).
6. Attribution for CFS Attribution Scale–The subject was asked to choose from 1 of 5 attributions (31):

a. My illness is a physical one.
b. My illness is mainly physical.
c. Both physical and psychological factors are involved with my illness.
d. My illness is mainly psychological.
e. My illness is psychological in nature.

RESULTS

An over all MANOVA was significant, Pillai Trace F (34, 62) = 2.2, p = .005, and a test for multi-colinearity showed that the personality variables are independent. Post-hoc tests for specific effects found significant differences for Alexithymia ($F(2, 51)$ = 5.8, p = 0.005), both MS (69 ± 2.9) and CFS (60 ± 2.3) were higher than Hea (54 ± 2.5). CFS was significantly lower on Health LOC measure for doctors/other control ($F(2, 51)$ = 8.6, p = 0.001) (Table 2). On the Attributional Style Questionnaire, both CFS and MS groups show significantly lower global attribution for good events ($F(2, 51)$ = 3.8, p = 0.03) and significantly higher stable attribution for bad events ($F(2,51)$ = 3.2, p = 0.04) compared to the healthy group (Table 3). There were no differences in perceived stress levels ($F(2, 51)$ = 1.1, p = 0.34) among the three groups

TABLE 2. Health Locus of Control

| | **Health Locus of Control** | | |
	Internal	Chance	Doctors/Others
CFS	17.8 ± 1.5	16.3 ± 1.5	$15.0 \pm 1.1^*$
MS	17.5 ± 1.6	18.0 ± 1.7	19.8 ± 1.2
HEA	22.4 ± 1.6	14.5 ± 1.3	21.1 ± 1.1

TABLE 3. Attributional Style

| | **Good Events** | | | **Bad Events** | | |
	Internal	Stable	Global	Internal	Stable	Global
CFS	5.2 ± 0.1	5.2 ± 0.2	4.6 ± 0.3	4.2 ± 0.2	4.2 ± 0.2	3.6 ± 0.3
MS	5.2 ± 0.4	5.4 ± 0.3	4.9 ± 0.3	4.5 ± 0.3	4.6 ± 0.3	3.7 ± 0.4
HEA	5.8 ± 0.3	5.3 ± 0.3	$5.2 \pm 0.4^*$	3.9 ± 0.4	$3.8 \pm 0.2^*$	3.5 ± 0.4

($^*p$ < .04, healthy significantly different from illness groups)

or on the hardiness measure which assessed challenge ($F(2, 51) = 2.7$, p = 0.08), control ($F(2, 51) = 1.6$, p = 0.21) and commitment ($F(2, 51) = 1.2$, p = 0.31) (Table 4). When CFS subjects were asked to choose an attribution for their illness, 43% selected the item "my illness is a physical one," 38% chose "my illness is mainly physical," while 19% elected "both physical and psychological factors are involved with my illness." No subjects chose psychological factors as predominant.

DISCUSSION

The finding of primarily physical attributions for CFS is redundant with a number of other studies showing them to be well defended psychologically with a tendency to minimize psychological contributions to their illness (22). This compares with Wessely & Powell's postviral fatigue syndrome patients in whom 86% attributed their fatigue to physical factors. In a prospective study of patients with viral illness, Cope et al. (32) found the tendency to attribute common symptoms to physical disorder rather than psychological factors or normal bodily responses was the most important risk factor for developing chronic post-viral fatigue. Studies examining illness behavior patterns (21,33,34), have found that CFS subjects tend to regard CFS as the sole problem in their lives, are resistant to psychological and social interpretations and maintain strong illness convictions. CFS patients strongly endorsed "a virus" or "pollution" as causes for their illness with "my own behavior" being the least favored attribution (34). However, a recent UK population-based incidence study of chronic fatigue, found that baseline fatigue score predicted subsequent chronic fatigue, and that when the confounding effects of fatigue levels were controlled psychological morbidity and physical attribution were not risk factors for chronic fatigue (35).

CFS and MS groups conveyed a more depressive attributional style than healthy participants, reflecting beliefs that causes for good events

TABLE 4. Hardiness Scale

	Challenge	Committment	Control	Total
CFS	35.7 ± 1.2	39.8 ± 0.7	38.4 ± 1.1	114 ± 2.2
MS	31.8 ± 1.9	38.0 ± 1.8	37.0 ± 1.9	107 ± 4.9
HEA	36.6 ± 1.5	41.5 ± 1.5	41.8 ± 1.7	121 ± 4.4

are not diffused into other areas of life while causes for bad events will always be present. This could reflect a development of learned helplessness in the face of uncertainty that characterizes the clinical course in both CFS and MS. The attributional style corroborates the HLOC results. Although both MS and CFS groups had lower internal LOC and higher ratings of the role of chance in events than the healthy group, these differences did not reach significance. It is likely that experience with chronic illness affects perceptions of control in that illness reduces control and chance likely plays a role in these illnesses. The genesis of illness is not controlled by individuals with MS or CFS, thus chance could be seen as a factor. CFS subjects scored significantly lower on Health Locus of Control for the doctors/others component than the MS or healthy groups, indicating lack of confidence or trust in medical professionals. This probably results from the lack of medical legitimacy awarded to CFS. The studies cited above indicate that CFS patients as a group espouse external explanations while rejecting purely psychological explanations. The patient is convinced that an organic etiology exists, while the biomedical community in failing to discover a consistent and convincing pathophysiology turns to psychiatry. Somatization patients also display chronic dissatisfaction with medical care, and often malign the diagnoses and therapies that physicians provide (36).

The personality variable of alexithymia in the CFS group resembles that of the MS group and both scored significantly higher than the healthy group on the Toronto Alexithymia Scale. Alexithymic behavior is hypothesized to predispose the individual to psychosomatic illness which occurs when the combination of physiological and cognitive responses to stress are disconnected (20). The MS patients scored highest on alexithymia, suggesting that chronic illness affects emotional regulation, even in patients having a disease with a known etiology. Results of the present study suggest that alexithymia could operate as a coping mechanism in chronic illness. Alexithymic tendencies could be protective against depression by preventing excessive internalization and rumination.

Alexithymia and antipathy towards medical professionals are important personality variables to be considered in future studies of CFS patients. These personality variables need to be recognized in order to enlist the patient in gaining some control over the symptoms of CFS and the effect that it has on their lives on a day to day basis. It would also benefit medical professionals in that patients with CFS could then better relay information on symptoms and various treatments to aid in defining and treating their disease.

Results indicate that CFS and MS are similar to each other while different from the healthy group on alexithymia and depressive attributional style which likely reflect the demoralizing effects of coping with a chronic, disabling illness marked by uncertainty. The CFS group was significantly lower on Doctors/Others LOC indicating lack of trust in medical professionals. When designating an attribution for CFS, 81% chose physical factors as primary, reflecting organic illness conviction and possible defensiveness regarding psychological views on the illness. CFS subjects have the additional burden of an illness that lacks medical legitimacy.

REFERENCES

1. Lane TJ, Manu P, Matthews DA: Depression and somatization in the chronic fatigue syndrome. Am J Med 1991; 91: 335-344.

2. Taerk GS, Toner BB, Salit IE, Garfinkel PE, Oersky S: Depression in patients with neuromyasthenia (benign myalgic encephalomyelitis). Intl J Psychiatry. 1987; 17: 49-56.

3. Wessely S, Chadler T, Hirsch S, Wallace P, Wright D: Psychological symptoms, somatic symptoms and psychiatric disorder in chronic fatigue and chronic fatigue syndrome: A prospective study in primary care. Am J Psychiatry 1996; 153: 1050-1059.

4. Millon C, Salvato F, Blaney N, Morgan R, Mantero-Atienza E, Klimas N, Fletcher M. A psychological assessment of chronic fatigue syndrome/chronic Epstein-Barr virus patients. Psychol and Health 1989; 3: 131-141.

5. Stricklin A, Sewell, M, Austad D. Objective measurement of personality variables in epidemic neuromyasthenia patients. S African Med J 1990; 77: 31-34.

6. Blakely AA, Howard RC, Sosich RM, Murdoch JC, Menkes DB, Spears GFS: Psychiatric symptoms, personality and ways of coping in chronic fatigue syndrome. Psychol Med 1991; 21: 347-362.

7. Pepper CM, Krupp LB, Friedberg F, Doscher C, Coyle PK: A comparison of neuropsychiatric characteristics in chronic fatigue syndrome, multiple sclerosis, and major depression. J Neuropsych and Clin Neurosci 1993; 5: 200-205.

8. Johnson, SK, DeLuca, J, Natelson, BH. Personality dimensions in CFS: A comparison with Multiple Sclerosis and depression. J Psychiatry Res 1996; 30: 1: 9-20.

9. Costa, PT, & McCrae, RR. Neuroticism, somatic complaints, and disease: Is the bark worse than the bite? J Personality 1987; 55: 299-316.

10. Zautra AJ, Okin MA, Robinson SE, LeeD, Roth SH, Emmanual J. Life stress and lymphocyte alterations among patients with rheumatoid arthritis. Health Psychol 1989; 8: 1-14.

11. Foley FW, Miller A, Traugott U, LaRocca NG, Scheinberg LC, Bedell JR, Lennox SS. Psychoimmunological dysregulation in multiple sclerosis. Psychosomatics 1988; 29: 398-403.

12. Grade M, Zegans LS. Exploring systemic lupus erythematosus: Autoimmunity, self-destruction, and psychoneuroimmunology. Advances 1986; 3: 16-45.

13. Kobasa SC. The hardy personality: Toward a social psychology of stress and health. In J Suls, G Sanders, & Erlbaum (Ed.), Social psychology of health and illness 1982; 3-33.

14. Burger JM. Negative reactions to increases in perceived personal control. J Pers and Soc Psychol 1989; 56: 246-256.

15. Hoehn-Saric R, McLeod DR. Locus of control in anxiety disorders. Acta Psychiatrica Scandanavica 1985; 72: 529-535.

16. Wallston KA, Stein M, Smith CA. Form C of the MHLC Scales: A condition specific measure of locus of control. J Pers Assess 1994; 63: 534-553.

17. Johnson SK, DeLuca J, Natelson: Depression in fatiguing illness: Comparing patients with chronic fatigue syndrome, multiple sclerosis and depression. J Affective Disorders 1996; 39: 21-30.

18. Huber S, Freidenberg D, Paulson G, Shuttleworth E, Christy J. The pattern of depressive symptoms varies with progression of Parkinson's disease. J Neurol Neurosurg Psychiatry 1990; 53: 275-278.

19. Peterson C, Seligman MEP. Explanatory style and illness. J Personality 1987; 55: 237-265.

20. Kohn PM, Gurevich M, Pickering DI, Macdonald JE. Alexithymia, reactivity, and the adverse impact of hassles-based stress. Personal Indiv Diffs 1994; 16: 6: 805-812.

21. Surawy C, Hackman A, Hawton K, Sharpe M. Chronic fatigue syndrome: A cognitive approach. Behavorial Research Therapy 1995; 33: 535-544.

22. Powell R, Dolan R, Wessely S. Attributions and self-esteem in depression and chronic fatigue syndrome. J Psychosomatic Research 1990; 21: 665-673.

23. Shorter E. Sucker-punched again! Physicians meet the disease of the month syndrome. J Psychiatric Research 1995; 39: 115-118.

24. Poser CM, Paty DW, Scheinberg L, McDonald WI, Davis FA, Ebers GC, Johnson, KP, Sibley WA, Silberberg DH, Tourtellotte WW. New diagnostic criteria for multiple sclerosis: Guidelines for research protocols. Ann Neurol 1988; 13: 227-231.

25. Holmes GP, Kaplan JE, Gantz NM, Komaroff AL, Schonberger LB, Straus SE, Jones JF, Dubois RE, Cunningham-Rundles C, Pahwa S, Tosato G, Zegans LS, Purtilo DT, Brown N, Schooley RT, Brus I. Chronic fatigue syndrome: A working case definition. Ann Internal Med 1988; 108: 387-389.

26. Schluederberg A, Straus SE, Peterson P, Blumenthal S, Komaroff AL, Spring SB, Landay A, Buchwald D. Chronic fatigue syndrome research. Definition and medical outcome assessment. Ann Internal Med 1992; 117: 325-331.

27. Cohen S, Kamarck T, Mermelstein R. A global measure of perceived stress. J Health & Soc Behav 1983; 24: 385-396.

28. Maddi SR, Kobasa, SC. The Hardy Executive: Health Under Stress 1984; Homewood, Ill: Dow Jones-Irwin.

29. Peterson C, Semmel A, Von Baeyer C, Abramson LY, Metalsky GI, Seligman MEP. The atrributional style questionnaire. Journal of Abnormal Psychology 1982; 6: 287-299.

30. Taylor GJ, Bagby RM, Ryan DP, Parker JDA, Doody KF, Keefe P. Criterion validity of the Toronto Alexithymia Scale. Psychosom Med 1988; 50: 500-509.

31. Wessely S, Powell R. Fatigue Syndrome: A comparison of chronic "post-viral" fatigue with neuromuscular and affective disorders. J Neurol Neurosurg Psychiatry 1989; 52: 940-949.

32. Cope H, David A, Pelosi A, Mann A. Predictors of chronic "post viral" fatigue. Lancet 1994; 344: 864-868.

33. Hickie I, Lloyd A, Wakefield D, Parker G. The psychiatric status of patients with chronic fatigue syndrome. Br J Psychiatry 1990; 156: 534-540.

34. Schweitzer R, Robertson DL, Kelly B, Whiting J. Illness behavior of patients with chronic fatigue syndrome. J Psychosom Res 1993; 38: 41-49.

35. Lawrie SM, Manders DN, Geddes JR, Pelosi AJ. A population-based incidence study of chronic fatigue. Psychol M\ed 1997; 27: 343-353.

36. Escobar JI. Transcultural aspects of dissociative and somatoform disorders. Cult Psychiat 1995; 18: 3: 555-569.

Chronic Fatigue Syndrome:
Overcoming the Attitudinal Impasse

E. Stein, MD FRCP(C)

SUMMARY. Context: Patients with Chronic Fatigue Syndrome and their physicians are often in conflict about the etiology and treatment of CFS.

Objectives: 1. Survey the literature regarding physician's attitudes towards CFS; 2. Examine the contributing factors to physician's attitude towards the disorder; and 3. Suggest solutions.

Data Sources: The relevant medical and psychological literature (years 1988-2000) was searched using the search term "Chronic Fatigue Syndrome." This was supplemented with papers from the bibliographies of the retrieved papers, additional related literature, and clinical experience.

Data Synthesis: Forty-six to ninety percent of GPs accept CFS as a discrete clinical entity and 30-82% are willing to make the diagnosis in qualifying patients.

Conclusions: CFS is a heterogeneous, multifactorial host response disorder that is inadequately described by the biomedical model. Despite substantial evidence of multisystemic physical abnormality in CFS, the lack of pathognomic tests and the female gender predominance cause

---

E. Stein is Staff Specialist in Psychiatry, Community Adolescent Team, The Junction, New South Wales. He is also Lecturer in Psychiatry, University of Newcastle, Callaghan, New South Wales.

Address correspondence to: E. Stein, c/o Community Adolescent Team, 36 Kenrick Street, The Junction, NSW, 2291 Australia (E-mail: aupsych@bigpond.com).

In memory of Dr. Naomi I. Rae Grant

The author would like to acknowledge the Collaborative Pain Research Unit, University of Newcastle and Allison Hunter Memorial Foundation.

[Haworth co-indexing entry note]: "Chronic Fatigue Syndrome: Overcoming the Attitudinal Impasse." Stein, E. Co-published simultaneously in *Journal of Chronic Fatigue Syndrome* (The Haworth Medical Press, an imprint of The Haworth Press, Inc.) Vol. 8, No. 3/4, 2001, pp. 53-61; and: *Innovations in Chronic Fatigue Syndrome Research and Clinical Practice* (ed: Roberto Patarca-Montero) The Haworth Medical Press, an imprint of The Haworth Press, Inc., 2001, pp. 53-61. Single or multiple copies of this article are available for a fee from The Haworth Document Delivery Service [1-800-342-9678, 9:00 a.m. - 5:00 p.m. (EST). E-mail address: getinfo@haworthpressinc.com].

some physicians to continue to treat CFS as a psychosocial disorder. This leads to conflict between patients and physicians. CFS challenges physicians to think beyond current disease models, to tolerate diagnostic and therapeutic uncertainty, and to work collaboratively with patients rather than taking the role of expert. *[Article copies available for a fee from The Haworth Document Delivery Service: 1-800-342-9678. E-mail address: <getinfo@haworthpressinc. com> Website: <http://www.HaworthPress.com> © 2001 by The Haworth Press, Inc. All rights reserved.]*

KEY WORDS. Attitudes, etiology, diagnosis

INTRODUCTION

Despite a large and growing evidence of immune, endocrine, autonomic and cognitive dysfunction in CFS, a precise understanding of CFS etiology and mechanism has not yet been reached (1). Inadequate definition, the heterogeneous presentation of patients with CFS and physician's discomfort with disorders which do not conform to a linear biomedical model have contributed to uncertainty among physicians as to the legitimacy of CFS as a discrete medical entity. Many physicians continue to formulate and treat CFS as a psychosocial disorder. Patients, on the other hand, believe their problems to be primarily of physical origin and are dissatisfied with treatment that does not address physical issues. The objective of this paper is to review the literature about physician's attitudes towards CFS, to examine the contributors to these attitudes and to suggest solutions to the current impasse

Quantitative data was gathered through a search of the literature (MEDLINE and PSYCHLIT 1988-2000) using the search term "Chronic Fatigue Syndrome" in it. All abstracts (n > 1500) were searched. The full text of all relevant papers was retrieved. The bibliographies of the retrieved papers and the full holdings of the *Journal of Chronic Fatigue Syndrome* (not in Medline) were searched by hand. This paper is not intended as a thorough review of the etiology or treatment of CFS but does include relevant examples to highlight useful conceptions and some of the common misconceptions about the disorder.

ACCEPTANCE OF CFS

The five published surveys of physician's attitudes towards CFS are summarized in Table 1. A sizable minority (10-54%) of GPs responding

TABLE 1. GPs acceptance of CFS

Study	Country	Selection method	Response rate (%)	Number of responding GPs	% Accepting existence of CFS	% Comfortable/able to diagnose CFS
Ho-Yen & McNamara 1991 (2)	2 counties, Scotland	total sample	91	178	71	n/a
Denz-Penhey et al. 1993 (3)	Otago New Zealand	total sample	85	97	90	69.5
Woodward et al. 1995 (4)	Canberra, Australia	solicited from GP branch	unclear	20	n/a	30
Fitzgibbon et al. 1997(5)	Ireland	random	72	118	58	82
Steven et al. 2000 (6)*	Australia	stratified by state	77	1615	46	66 (made dx in past year)

* survey completed in 1995 but not reported until 2000
n/a–not reported

to the surveys are uncomfortable with the concept of CFS as a clinical entity. As few as thirty percent of responding GPs were willing to diagnose CFS in patients meeting the criteria. It is likely that among the survey non-respondents acceptance of CFS is even lower. The acceptance rates may not seem inordinately low. However, if other disorders of unknown etiology (e.g., multiple sclerosis, rheumatoid arthritis) were substituted for CFS non-acceptance by even a small percentage of practicing GPs would be unacceptable.

Of the physicians who remain reluctant to make the diagnosis of CFS, some argue that it is unethical to diagnose a disorder which cannot be treated (3) while others worry that a diagnosis of CFS will encourage illness behavior that will perpetuate disability (5). There is no research evidence to support this concern. In fact the opposite may be true. Patients without a firm diagnosis may seek further opinions (3). Unfortunately some physicians shy away from diagnosing and treating CFS in order to avoid controversy or scrutiny from their peers (3).

PATIENT-PHYSICIAN CONFLICT

At the core of the conflict between physicians and patients lies disparate views about the etiology of CFS. Most patients cite physical factors as the primary cause of their illness (6). Physicians, on the other hand, feel uncomfortable assuming a physical cause when no precise physical etiology has been established. Dissatisfaction and conflict between patients and their physicians is more common with CFS than with other chronic medical disorders (7). Patients with CFS report that their concerns are not taken seriously and that they are not given the emotional or informational support that they need (7-9). Physicians express frustration with the quality of care they provide patients with CFS (4). They report that patients with CFS take up extra time during consultations (1) and are "difficult" to treat (10,11). This is especially true for patients who have self-diagnosed with CFS (9,10). Although the conflict between patients with CFS and their physicians is predicated upon the lack of legitimacy of CFS, both physicians and patients tend to blame each other.

CFS IS NOT YET WELL DEFINED

Part of the problem arises from inadequate definition of CFS. There are four definitions currently in use. Each is the result of clinical experience and consensus and as such reflects the assumptions of the creators. For example, the most stringent criteria (CDC 1988) require both physical symptoms and signs in addition to disabling, prolonged fatigue (12) whereas the least stringent (Oxford, Australian) require neither (13,14). The most widely used definition (CDC 1994) for CFS requires the concurrent expression for at least 6 months of fatigue that substantially limits functioning and is accompanied by at least four of the following symptoms: post-exertional fatigue, muscle or joint pain, cognitive changes, axillary or cervical lymphadenopathy, headache, sore throat and sleep disturbance (15). However, most patients report additional symptoms which are not included in any of the above definitions, e.g., visual blurring, clumsiness, parasthesias, paralysis, nocturia, nausea, orthostatic intolerance, alcohol intolerance, gastrointestinal and sicca symptoms. (13,16-18)

A factor analysis of the largest CFS patient set yet reported (n = 1573) confirms heterogeneity. CFS consists of three different independent factor groupings: immune/general, cognitive and musculoskeletal (19). Each of these three factor groups differentiated between defined CFS patients and controls. A fourth factor grouping of emotional/psychiatric symptoms failed to discriminate. This suggests that the current definitions need to be revised to: include more discriminating symptoms, consider multiple symptom dimensions and to decrease the emphasis currently given to psychiatric disorder.

CFS IS A MISLEADING LABEL

Many argue that the label "Chronic Fatigue Syndrome" contributes to the disorder's lack of legitimacy because it emphasizes only one symptom "fatigue," which is such a common and non-specific symptom. The name fails to convey that the mental and physical fatigue in CFS are not substantially relieved by rest nor that exertion worsens symptoms. The lack of mention of physical signs and symptoms in the label allows the inclusion of a very heterogeneous group of less severely ill patients to be considered under the rubric of CFS. As a result many research hypotheses and findings may not pertain to patients with tightly defined CFS who have multisystemic involvement.

CFS AND THE MEDICAL MODEL

The medical model encourages physicians to examine patients for signs and symptoms, make a diagnosis and then implement diagnosis based treatment. Although not explicit in the medical model, it is usually assumed that specific genetic or external factors result in specific clinical presentations in a linear fashion. Disorders such as CFS which are non-specific host responses to unknown or multiple stressors fit poorly into a biomedical model. It cannot be overemphasized that there is nothing inherent in the medical model that makes it ill suited to conditions such as CFS. Indeed, bio-psycho-social formulations for all medical presentations are encouraged. However, these holistic formulations are difficult to implement in a busy general medical practice (21).

Early skeptics of the validity of CFS (then referred to as benign myalgic encephalomyelitis) cite the female preponderance of sufferers and the lack of definitive physical findings as evidence that the disorder was hysterical in nature (21). Similar logic informs recent papers espousing a psychosocial etiology for CFS. The thesis of this paper is that absence of evidence does not constitute evidence of absence. Medical history is replete with incorrect assumptions of psychological etiology prior to technology becoming available to prove otherwise. Schizophrenia, multiple sclerosis, peptic ulcer disease, inflammatory bowel disease, asthma, tuberculosis and myasthenia gravis are only a few examples.

PHYSICIAN'S DISCOMFORT WITH UNCERTAINTY

It is a puzzle why so many physicians are reluctant to admit that CFS is a valid and debilitating disorder that has not yet been adequately described. Up to 80% of patients presenting to general practitioners cannot be given a diagnostic label that fully accounts for their symptoms (22,23). Being uncertain of diagnosis or treatment is certainly unsettling for physicians and can lead to feelings of helplessness and incompetence. The greater the discomfort, the more likely physicians are to jump to conclusions based on partial evidence. This is especially true when the incorrect conclusions are supported by colleagues held in high esteem. The pressure from health service funders for rapid diagnosis and treatment places additional pressure on physicians to make premature and simplistic conclusions.

OVERCOMING THE IMPASSE

A respectful and collaborative approach to CFS management requires physicians to maintain a healthy skepticism of what they have learnt. Current medical knowledge cannot adequately explain CFS. When patients present with symptoms that seem "impossible" or "bizarre," physicians must be willing to question both their patients and their medical knowledge. Instead of assuming that the patient is mistaken or neurotic, physicians must try to explain what they see and resist the temptation of simplistic explanations even when they come from reputable sources.

In many cases, frustrations within the doctor-patient relationship are a result of conflicting views about CFS etiology and treatment. It is important to remember that such conflicts are relational or contextual issues and not necessarily suggestive of either patient or physician psychopathology.

Management should be aimed at supporting healthy body functioning and treatment of symptoms that contribute to morbidity. Each symptom is understood in the context of its function and its relation to the rest of the body. Some of the ancillary symptoms found in CFS are treatable, e.g., postural hypotension (24), hypocortisolemia (25), psychiatric disorder, irritable bowel syndrome (26), bacterial infection (27) and irritable bowel symptoms (26). Although treating concomitant disorders rarely "cures" CFS, it may decrease patient morbidity.

Because there is no gold standard for CFS treatment, physicians and patients must share the responsibility for information gathering and monitoring of the patient's progress. Each patient becomes an N = 1 experiment in which the observations of both patient and physician inform critical decision making. Asking patients to keep daily symptom diaries and then reviewing symptom ratings before and after treatment trials is a powerful way of assessing outcome. Few patients will choose to pursue a harmful or ineffective treatment in the face of their own conflicting evidence.

CONCLUSION

The medical profession is at a crossroads. Approaching a problem repeatedly in the same manner generally leads to predictable results. If physicians continue to assume patients with CFS are psychologically disturbed just because medical technology cannot yet explain the physical aspects of their disorder, it is likely that the current discontent between patients with CFS and physicians will continue. Alternatively, accepting ignorance as an inevitable and challenging aspect of medicine will enable physicians to work with patients to discover the causes and mechanisms of CFS and may herald a new approach to multifaceted disorders such as CFS that are not yet well understood.

REFERENCES

1. Komaroff AL. The biology of chronic fatigue syndrome. American Journal of Medicine 2000; 108: 169-171.

2. Ho-Yen DO, McNamara I. General practitioner's experience of the chronic fatigue syndrome. British Journal of General Practice 1991; 41 (349): 324-326.

3. Denz-Penhey H, Murdoch JC. General practitioners acceptance of the validity of chronic fatigue syndrome as a diagnosis. New Zealand Medical Journal 1993; 106 (953): 122-124.

4. Woodward RV, Broom DH, Legge DG. Diagnosis in chronic illness: disabling or enabling–the case of chronic fatigue syndrome. Journal of the Royal Society of Medicine 1995; 88 (6): 325-329.

5. Fitzgibbon EJ, Murphy D, O'Shea K, Kelleher C. Chronic debilitating fatigue in Irish general practice: a survey of general practitioner's experience. British Journal of General Practice 1997; 47 (423): 618-622.

6. Steven ID, McGrath B, Qureshi F, Wong C, Chern I, Pern-Rowe B. General Practitioner's beliefs, attitudes and reported actions towards chronic fatigue syndrome. Australian Family Physician 2000; 29 (1): 80-85.

7. Sharpe M, Hawton K, Simkin S, Surawy C, Hackmann A, Klimes I et al. Cognitive behavior therapy for the chronic fatigue syndrome: a randomized controlled trial. BMJ 1996; 312 (7022): 22-26.

8. Twemlow SW, Bradshaw SL, Jr., Coyne L, Lerma BH. Patterns of utilization of medical care and perceptions of the relationship between doctor and patient with chronic illness including chronic fatigue syndrome. Psychological Reports 1997; 80 (2): 643-658.

9. Ax S, Gregg VH, Jones D. Chronic fatigue syndrome: sufferer's evaluation of medical support. Journal of the Royal Society of Medicine 1997; 90 (5): 250-254.

10. Green J, Romei J, Natelson BH. Stigma and chronic fatigue syndrome. Journal of Chronic Fatigue Syndrome 1999; 5 (2): 63-76.

11. Scott S, Deary I, Pelosi AJ. General practitioner's attitudes to patients with a self diagnosis of myalgic encephalomyelitis. BMJ 1995; 310 (6978): 508.

12. Sharpe M, Mayou R, Seagroatt V, Surawy C, Warwick H, Bulstrode C et al. Why do doctors find some patients difficult to help? Q J Med 1994; 87 (3): 187-193.

13. Holmes GP, Kaplan JE, Gantz NM, Komaroff AL, Schonberger LB, Straus SE et al. Chronic fatigue syndrome: a working case definition. Annals of Internal Medicine 1988; 108 (3): 387-389.

14. Lloyd AR, Hickie I, Boughton CR, Spencer O, Wakefield D. Prevalence of chronic fatigue syndrome in an Australian population. The Medical Journal of Australia 1990; 153: 522-528.

15. Sharpe MC, Archard LC, Banatvala JE, Borysiewicz LK, Clare AW, David A et al. A report–chronic fatigue syndrome: guidelines for research. Journal of the Royal Society of Medicine 1991; 84: 118-121.

16. Fukuda K, Straus SE, Hickie I, Sharpe MC, Dobbins JG, Komaroff A et al. The chronic fatigue syndrome: a comprehensive approach to its definition and study. Annals of Internal Medicine 1994; 121 (12): 953-959.

17. Komaroff AL, Buchwald D. Symptoms and Signs of Chronic Fatigue Syndrome. RID 1991; 13 (Suppl 1): S8-S11.

18. Friedberg F, Dechene L, McKenzie MJ, Fontanetta R. Symptom patterns in long-duration chronic fatigue syndrome. Journal of Psychosomatic Research 2000; 48 (1): 59-68.

19. Smith AP, Borysiewicz L, Pollock J, Thomas M, Perry K, Llewelyn M. Acute fatigue in chronic fatigue syndrome patients. Psychological Medicine 1999; 29 (2): 283-290.

20. De Becker P, McGregor NR, De Meirleir K. A factor analysis study of symptoms in 1573 patients with chronic fatigue syndrome. Vrije Universiteit Brussel, 2000.

21. Straus SE. Chronic fatigue syndrome. BMJ 1996; 313 (7061): 831-832.

22. McEvedy CP, Beard AW. Royal Free Epidemic of 1955: A reconsideration. BMJ 1970; 1: 7-11.

23. Kroenke K, Mangelsdorff AD. Common symptoms in ambulatory care: incidence, evaluation, therapy, and outcome. American Journal of Medicine 1989; 86 (3): 262-266.

24. Bridges-Webb C, Britt H, Miles D, Neary S, Charles J, Traynor V. Morbidity and treatment in general practice in Australia 1990-1991. Medical Journal of Australia 1992; 157: S1-S53.

25. Bou-Holaigah I, Rowe PC, Kan J, Calkins H. The relationship between neurally mediated hypotension and the chronic fatigue syndrome. JAMA 1995; 274 (12): 961-967.

26. Cleare AJ, Heap E, Malhi GS, Wessely S, O'Keane V, Miell J. Low-dose hydrocortisone in chronic fatigue syndrome: a randomised crossover trial. Lancet 1999; 353 (9151): 455-458.

27. Paterson WG, Thompson WG, Vanner SJ, Faloon TR, Rosser WW, Birtwhistle et al. Recommendations for the management of irritable bowel syndrome in family practice. IBS Consensus Conference Participants. CMAJ 1999; 161 (2): 154-160.

28. Nicolson GL, Nasralla MY, Haier J, Irwin R, Nicolson NL, Ngwenya R. Mycoplasmal infections in chronic illnesses: fibromyalgia and chronic fatigue syndromes, gulf war illness, HIV-AIDS and rheumatoid arthritis. Medical Sentinal 1999; 4 (5): 172-191.

G-Actin Cleavage Parallels 2-5A-Dependent RNase L Cleavage in Peripheral Blood Mononuclear Cells– Relevance to a Possible Serum-Based Screening Test for Dysregulations in the 2-5A Pathway

Simon Roelens, MS
C. Vincent Herst, PhD
Anne D'Haese, MS
Karen De Smet, PhD
Marc Frémont, PhD
Kenny De Meirleir, MD, PhD
Patrick Englebienne, PhD

Simon Roelens, C. Vincent Herst, Anne D'Haese, Karen De Smet and Marc Frémont are affiliated with RED Laboratories, N.V., Brussels, Belgium.

Kenny De Meirleir is affiliated with the Vrije Universiteit Brussel, Brussels, Belgium.

Patrick Englebienne is affiliated with the Université Libre de Bruxelles (Brugmann Hospital) and is Consultant, RED Laboratories, Brussels, Belgium.

Address correspondence to: Dr. Patrick Englebienne, RED Laboratories, N.V., Pontbeek 61, B-1731 Zellik, Belgium (E-mail: penglebienne@redlabs.be).

[Haworth co-indexing entry note]: "G-Actin Cleavage Parallels 2-5A-Dependent RNase L Cleavage in Peripheral Blood Mononuclear Cells–Relevance to a Possible Serum-Based Screening Test for Dysregulations in the 2-5A Pathway." Roelens, Simon et al. Co-published simultaneously in *Journal of Chronic Fatigue Syndrome* (The Haworth Medical Press, an imprint of The Haworth Press, Inc.) Vol. 8, No. 3/4, 2001, pp. 63-82; and: *Innovations in Chronic Fatigue Syndrome Research and Clinical Practice* (ed: Roberto Patarca-Montero) The Haworth Medical Press, an imprint of The Haworth Press, Inc., 2001, pp. 63-82. Single or multiple copies of this article are available for a fee from The Haworth Document Delivery Service [1-800-342-9678, 9:00 a.m. - 5:00 p.m. (EST). E-mail address: getinfo@haworthpressinc.com].

SUMMARY. A dysregulation in the 2′,5′-oligoadenylate (2-5A)-dependent RNase L antiviral pathway has been detected in peripheral blood mononuclear cells (PBMC) of chronic fatigue syndrome (CFS) patients, which is characterized by an unregulated RNase L activity and the presence of a low molecular weight (LMW) 2-5A-binding protein (37-kDa 2-5A-BP). This study was undertaken to test the possibility that the 37-kDa 2-5A-BP of CFS is produced by proteolytic cleavage of the 80-kDa monomeric enzyme. Incubation of the 80-kDa human recombinant RNase L (r-hRNase L) with PBMC extracts either positive or negative for the presence of 37-kDa 2-5A-BP, respectively, demonstrates that the LMW protein is produced by the former, not the latter, and that the size of the fragment generated from the recombinant protein matches the 37-kDa size of the fragment observed in the original PBMC. Digestion of r-hRNase L with calpain generated the same 37-kDa 2-5A-BP observed in PBMC extracts, and calpain immunoprecipitation from PBMC extracts reduced their proteolytic activity, an observation that suggests that calpain may be involved in the cleavage. We further examined G-actin, a known calpain substrate, for possible cleavage in PBMC. Actin fragments were observed of which the presence correlated with the presence of 37-kDa 2-5-BP. Since G-actin is cleared by serum transport, we further screened serum samples for the presence of LMW forms. A single LMW actin fragment could be detected in serum, the presence of which correlated significantly with the presence of both G-actin and RNase L fragments in PBMC. This latter observation offers the opportunity to screen large populations of patients for dysregulations in the RNase L pathway by a serum-based assay. *[Article copies available for a fee from The Haworth Document Delivery Service: 1-800-342-9678. E-mail address: <getinfo@haworthpressinc.com> Website: <http://www.HaworthPress. com> © 2001 by The Haworth Press, Inc. All rights reserved.]*

KEYWORDS. G-Actin, RNase L, 37-kDa 2-5A-binding protein, chronic fatigue syndrome, CFS, serum screening test, apoptosis, PBMC, 2-5A pathway, calpain

INTRODUCTION

The interferon (IFN)-inducible 2′,5′-oligoadenylate (2-5A) synthetase/ribonuclease L (RNase L) pathway is involved in eukaryotic cell protection against viruses. IFN triggers the production of nearly micromolar concentrations of 2-5A by virus-infected cells (1). The 2-5A are generated from ATP by any of several isozymes of an 2-5A synthetase specifically activated by double-stranded RNA of viral origin (2). The regulation by IFN of the 2-5A anti-viral mechanisms involves also the enhanced expression of an 2-5A-dependent RNase, termed RNase L. This 80 kDa monomeric latent protein is activated by binding 2-5A and homodimerizes during this activation process (3). The activated dimeric enzyme cleaves single-stranded RNA of viral and cellular origin, primarily after UpNp sequences (4), which results in the inhibition of protein synthesis.

Chronic fatigue syndrome (CFS) is a poorly understood physical condition defined exclusively by a group of symptoms listed in the case definition developed by the Centers for Disease Control and Prevention (reviewed in 5). Typically, the onset of CFS is sudden, often with a flu-like illness, and an accumulating body of evidence suggests that CFS results from a dysregulation of both humoral (6) and cellular (7) immunity. Several causes have been suggested for the onset and maintenance of the disease, including the reactivation of hidden viral infections (8). However, subsequent studies demonstrated that this etiology could not be generalized (9). Recently, an increased sensitivity to glucocorticoids has been proposed as the origin for the altered immune function of CFS (10).

Early on, a severe dysregulation in the key components of the 2-5A pathway had been evidenced in CFS (11,12) and more recently (13), a LMW 37-kDa 2-5A binding RNase L form (37-kDa 2-5A-BP) has been identified in the peripheral blood mononuclear cells (PBMC) of CFS patients. Further to this latter finding, the 37-kDa 2-5A-BP has been proposed as a possible biochemical marker for CFS (14). Whilst proteolytic degradation of the 80-kDa native enzyme has been suggested as a possible origin for the LMW form (13), no definitive evidence has so far been provided. Using a recombinant human RNase L (r-hRNase L), we show in this report that the LMW form present in CFS PBMC arises by proteolytic cleavage of the 80-kDa monomeric enzyme. Moreover, we show that G-actin, a calpain substrate is also cleaved in CFS PBMC and the presence of actin fragments correlates with the presence of RNase L fragments. These data further support the involvement of an increased rate of immune cell apoptosis in the onset and maintenance of the disease (15). Because G-actin is cleared from damaged cells by serum transport (16), we looked for the presence of fragments in serum and report here that the presence of a G-actin fragment in serum correlates significantly with the presence of both G-actin and RNase L fragments in PBMC. We finally suggest to use the detection of G-actin fragment in serum as a screening test for dysregulations in the 2-5A pathway, which would eventually be confirmed by the detection of the 37-kDa 2-5A-BP in PBMC (14).

MATERIALS AND METHODS

Study Subjects and Samples

Study subjects were individuals selected from a medical practice at the University of Brussels for analysis of the 37-kDa 2-5A-BP in PBMC as previously described (14). At the time of heparinized blood draw for PBMC preparation, a serum separator tube was also collected for other routine tests. Portions of samples remaining after the routine assays had been performed and validated were used in this study.

Peripheral Blood Mononuclear Cells (PBMC), Cell Extracts and Serum

PBMC were separated from heparinized blood (30 ml) by Ficoll-Hypaque density gradient centrifugation within four hours of blood draw as previously described (11). The PBMCs were then stored at $-70°C$ until cytoplasmic extracts could be made. Cytoplasmic extracts were prepared in the presence of the protease inhibitors aprotinin, leupeptin, pefabloc-SC and EDTA (Roche Biochemicals, Mannheim, Germany) as previously described (11). Serum was separated from co-agulated blood in the same timeframe according to standard laboratory procedures and stored at $-70°C$ until analyzed.

Quantification of total proteins in the patient cell extracts and serum was performed using a modified Bradford assay method (Bio-Rad Laboratories, Hercules, CA) according to the manufacturer's procedure.

Quantification of 37-kDa 2-5A-BP in PBMC Extracts

Analysis was performed by sodium dodecylsulfate polyacrylamide gel electrophoresis (SDS-PAGE), using a metaperiodate (10 mM final concentration, pH 4.75) oxidized 2-5A trimer radiolabeled at the 3′ end with ^{32}P-pCp as the reporter ligand (14). Briefly, the radiolabeled 2-5A trimer was incubated with 200 µg of cell extract at 2-4°C for 15 minutes to allow for interaction with any 2-5A-BP present and was then covalently attached to the binding proteins by the addition of cyanoborohydride (20 mM in 100 mM phosphate buffer, pH 8.0). The reduction reaction was allowed to occur for 20 minutes at 2-4°C. SDS-PAGE buffer, including a tracking dye, was added to the samples which were incubated at 95°C for 5 minutes. The samples were then subjected to standard SDS-PAGE using a 4% stacking and a 10% separating gel. The gel was then dried and subjected to autoradiography (Bio-Rad Laboratories Molecular Imager® Fx, Hercules, CA). The autoradiographs were analyzed by densitometry, and quantification of any 2-5A-BP present was performed using a specialized software (Quantity One® Software from Bio-Rad Laboratories, Hercules, CA). The results were expressed as the percentage of 80-kDa native RNase L present in the sample (80-kDa/[80-kDa + 37-kDa] $\times$ 100).

Production of Recombinant Human RNase L Protein

r-hRNaseL was cloned, and expressed in baculovirus transfected Sf21 insect cells by ATG Laboratories (Eden Prairie, MN). An His6-tag was inserted at the aminoterminus of the protein which was purified to 90-95% homogeneity by metal chelate chromatography on Ni-Nitrilo-triacetic acid-agarose. A monoclonal antibody raised against tetra-histidine (Qiagen, Venlo, The Netherlands) specifically recognizes a single band in the purified protein solution with an apparent molecular weight of 84-kDa by SDS-PAGE.

In Vitro Cleavage of r-hRNase L by PBMC Extracts, Caspase-3 and Calpain

The radiolabeled 2-5A probe was incubated with 10 μg of r-hRNase L at 2-4°C for 15 minutes. The bound radiolabeled 2-5A was then covalently attached by the addition of cyanoborohydride as described above. *In vitro* cleavage of r-hRNase L radiolabeled with 2-5A was then performed by incubating 295 ng of protein at 37°C during the times indicated with either 2 μg of PBMC proteins, 2 or 5 units of purified caspase-3 (BioSource International, Nivelles, Belgium) or 0.42 unit of neutral calcium activated protease (calpain, Sigma, St. Louis, MO), respectively, previously preincubated during 30 min at 37°C in the presence or absence of the inhibitors (caspase-3 inhibitor Z-DEVD-Fmk from Calbiochem, Bad Soden, Germany; calpain inhibitor I and II, N-Ac-LLnorleucinal and N-Ac-LLmethioninal, respectively, from Roche Biochemicals, Mannheim, Germany; PD150607 or calpastatin from

Calbiochem). Where indicated, prior to their incubation with the labeled r-hRNase L, the cell extracts were incubated with anti-calpain antibodies during one hour at 4°C (anti m-calpain C268 and anti μ-calpain C267 from Sigma, St. Louis, MO at 1:10 v:v dilution in extraction buffer) and the complexes were immunoprecipitated with protein A Sepharose (Amersham-Pharmacia Biotech, Amersham, UK). Proteins were then resolved by SDS-PAGE and the labeled polypeptides were detected by autoradiography as described above. The inhibition of proteolysis in the presence of inhibitors was expressed as the increase in percentage of the 80-kDa r-hRNase L measured by densitometry as described above.

Immunoblotting Analysis of G-Actin and Its Fragments in PBMC Extracts and Serum

To analyze PBMC extracts and serum for the presence of G-actin and related fragments, either 200 μg of PBMC or 250 μg of serum proteins were subjected to standard SDS-PAGE using a 12.5% separating gel. The separated proteins were then transferred to a 0.2 μm PVDF membrane (Bio-Rad Laboratories, Hercules, CA) using a semi-dry transfer system (Amersham-Pharmacia Biotech, Amersham, UK). Transfer was performed at an average current of 0.8 mA per cm^2 for two hours. After transfer was complete, the membrane was allowed to dry thoroughly at room temperature for at least one hour. The membrane was then wet with a minimum volume of 100% methanol, subsequently replaced by a solution of 5% (w:v) non-fat dry milk in phosphate-buffered saline, pH 7.4 containing 0.1% (v:v) Tween 20 (PBS-Tween) as blocking buffer, and the membrane was incubated for one hour with gentle shaking. The blocking buffer was discarded and fresh blocking buffer containing the primary antibody (1:500 v:v dilution in PBS of rabbit G-actin polyclonal antibodies directed against the N-, cat. A 5060, or C-terminal end of G-actin, cat. A 2066 from Sigma, St. Louis, MO). The membrane was allowed to react with the antibody for two hours with gentle shaking. The primary antibody solution was then discarded and the membrane was washed three times with 25 ml PBS-Tween. After the last wash, fresh blocking buffer containing the secondary antibody at 1:3,000 v:v dilution (goat anti-rabbit antibody conjugated to horseradish peroxidase from Bio-Rad Laboratories, Hercules, CA) was added and the membrane was incubated for 30 min with gentle shaking. The secondary antibody solution was discarded and the membrane was washed three times with 25 ml PBS-Tween. Color development was then performed using the Opti4-CN® kit from Bio-Rad Laboratories (Hercules, CA), and the proteins detected were quantified by densitometry as described above. The results were expressed as the percentage of native monomeric G-actin present as related to the total immunoreactive actin species detected.

In Vitro Cleavage of G-Actin by Caspase-3 and Calpain

In vitro cleavage of purified human G-actin (Cytoskeleton, Denver, CO) was performed by incubating 2 μg of protein with either purified caspase-3 (2 or 8 units) or calpain (0.25 or 1.5 units) for 1 or 6 hours at 37°C, previously preincubated in presence or absence of the inhibitors. Proteins were then separated by 12.5% SDS-PAGE and immunoblotting analysis was performed as described above.

RESULTS

The 37-kDa RNase L Arises from Proteolytic Cleavage of the Native 80-kDa Enzyme

PBMC extracts from CFS patients are characterized by the presence of a 37-kDa 2-5A-BP that can be identified, along with the 80-kDa monomeric RNase L, after incubation of the samples with radioactive 2-5A and subsequent SDS-PAGE in reducing conditions (14). As shown on Figure 1A, the 37-kDa 2-5A-BP is more or less present in different samples and the more the 37-kDa 2-5A-BP is present, the less the 80-kDa monomeric RNase L can be detected (compare Figure 1A, lanes 1 to 3). This is likely to suggest that the 37-kDa protein originates from the 80-kDa native enzyme by proteolytic cleavage. In order to verify this hypothesis, the 80-kDa human RNase L cDNA sequence (17) was cloned, expressed in Sf21 insect cells and the His-tagged protein purified by affinity chromatography was used as a substrate to investigate the proteolytic activity of PBMC extracts. The protein was covalently labeled with the radioactive 2-5A probe and incubated with either PBMC extracts or purified enzymes, respectively, and subjected to SDS-PAGE in reducing conditions. The labeled bands were then identified by autoradiography. As shown in Figure 1B, incubation during 5, 15 and 30 min of the labeled r-hRNase L, respectively, with PBMC extracts ei-

FIGURE 1. The 37-kDa 2-5A-BP is produced by proteolytic cleavage of the 80-kDa RNase L. Calpain, but not caspase-3, is one possible protease involved in the cleavage

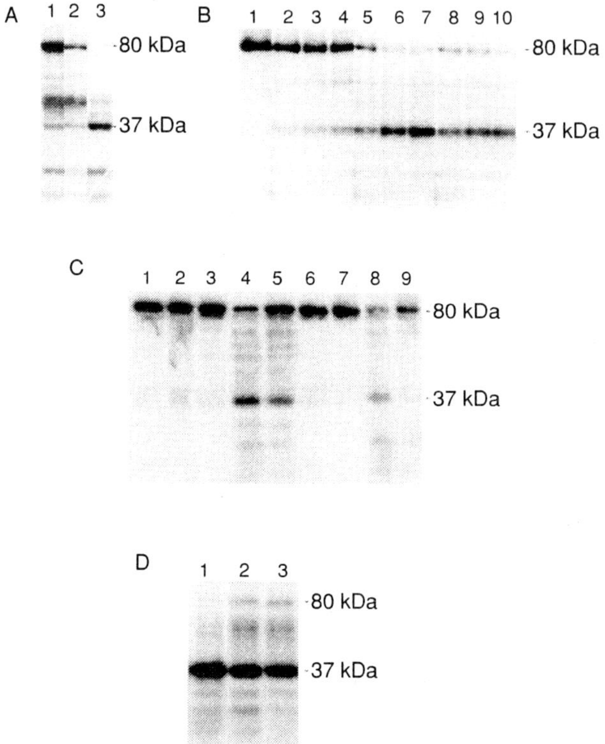

A. CFS PBMC extracts incubated and labeled with radioactive 2-5A were subjected to SDS-PAGE and subsequent autoradiography, so as to identify the native 2-5A-binding proteins, including the 37-kDa 2-5A-BP and the 80-kDa RNase L. The PBMC samples shown are progressively positive (from lane 1 to lane 3) for the presence of the 37-kDa 2-5A-BP. The progressive presence of the 37-kDa protein is paralleled by a progressive decrease in the 80-kDa monomeric RNase L which suggests that the former originates from the proteolytic cleavage of the latter.

B. r-hRNase L was labeled with the 2-5A radioactive probe and incubated during either 30 min at 37°C with buffer (control, lane 1) or during 5, 15 and 30 min. at 37°C with PBMC extracts either negative (lanes 2-4) or positive (lanes 5-7 and 8-10) for the presence of 37-kDa 2-5A-BP, and then analyzed by SDS-PAGE and autoradiography. Incubation of the recombinant protein with the positive extracts progressively leads to the disappearance of the 80-kDa monomer, which is concommittant to the appearance of the 37-kDa fragment.

C. The labeled r-hRNase L (control lane 1) was, respectively, incubated during 30 min. at 37°C with 2 and 5 units of caspase-3 (lanes 2 and 3, respectively), 0.42 units of calpain (lane 4), calpain and caspase-3 (lane 5), caspase-3 in presence of 1 or 5 nM of caspase inhibitor (lanes 6 and 7, respectively), or calpain in presence of 200 or 400 nM of calpain inhibitor I (lanes 8 and 9, respectively). Caspase-3 fails to cleave the protein, whilst calpain generates the 37-kDa 2-5A-BP from the 80-kDa enzyme and the process is blocked in the presence of calpain inhibitor I.

D. The labeled r-hRNase L was incubated during 30 min at 37°C with one PBMC extract positive for the presence of 37-kDa 2-5A-BP either untreated (lane 1) or immunoprecipitated with antibodies specific for m-(lane 2) and μ-calpain (lane 3), respectively, before being analyzed by SDS-PAGE and autoradiography. Failure to block fully the proteolytic activity of the PBMC extracts after calpain removal by immunoprecipitation suggests the involvement of other protease(s).

ther positive (lanes 5-10) or negative (lanes 2-4) for the presence of the 37-kDa 2-5A-BP led to the progressive formation of a 37-kDa fragment with the positive extracts only. The fragment produced from the recombinant enzyme had exactly the same size as the 37-kDa protein present in the PBMC extracts (compare with Figure 1A).

Because the PBMC extracts were prepared in the presence of inhibitors for the most common protease families, we turned toward the apoptotic proteases caspase-3 (18) and calpain (19) as possible actors for the cleavage. Figure 1B demonstrates that calpain (lane 4-5), not the caspase (lanes 2-3 and 6-7), cleaved the recombinant enzyme, generating a 37-kDa 2-5A-BP of the same size as that found in the positive PBMC extracts (Figure 1A). Moreover, the cleavage by pure calpain was reduced in the presence of a specific inhibitor (Figure 1C, lanes 8 and 9). When the labeled r-hRNase L was incubated with an extract positive for the presence of 37-kDa 2-5A-BP (Figure 1D, lane 1), the formation of the 37-kDa fragment was reduced and more 80-kDa RNase L could be detected when the incubation occured after the calpain had been removed by immunoprecipitation with antibodies specific for both μ- and m-calpain (Figure 1D, lanes 2 and 3), respectively. As shown in Figure 2, a reduction of the proteolytic activity was also observed when the incubation of PBMC extracts with r-hRNase L was carried out in presence of four calpain inhibitors at two different concentrations. The extent of proteolytic inhibition varied from 2 to 39%, depending on the original proteolytic activity of the extract (% of 80-kDa RNase L in absence of inhibitor) and on the inhibitor used. Only PBMC extracts possessing a medium or high proteolytic activity were significantly inhibited by the calpain inhibitors.

The Presence of LMW G-Actin Fragments Correlates with the Presence of 37-kDa 2-5A-BP in PBMC

Further to the observation we had made that the 37-kDa 2-5A-BP was likely to be produced by calpain cleavage of the 80-kDa RNase L in PBMC, we looked at other cellular proteins that could be cleaved by the same enzyme. Among the apoptotic substrates, G-actin is likely to play a pivotal role (20) and we screened PBMC extracts that had been analyzed for the 37-kDa 2-5A-BP for the presence of G-actin fragments by immunoblotting. For the detection, we used two different antibodies specific for either the N- or C-terminal portions of G-actin. Figure 3 displays a representative example of such a blot. Both antibodies detected

FIGURE 2. Inhibition of the proteolytic activity of PBMC extracts by calpain inhibitors, either calpastatin (part A), PD 150607 (part B), calpain inhibitors I (part C) and II (part D). r-hRNase L was labeled with the 2-5A radioactive probe and incubated during 15 min at 37°C with the extracts, respectively, in absence or presence of the inhibitors at two different concentrations and then submitted to SDS-PAGE and autoradiography. The original proteolytic activity of the three samples was rated by their ability to cleave the recombinant protein in the absence of the inhibitors, as expressed by the percentage of the 80-kDa band over the sum of 80 + 37-kDa bands remaining after incubation. The original proteolytic activities were low (72% 80-kDa RNase L, crosses), medium (63% 80-kDa RNase L, triangles) and high (27% 80-kDa RNase L, circles). The inhibition of the proteolytic activity in presence of the different inhibitors was expressed by the increase in the percentage of 80-kDa RNase L measured after incubation.

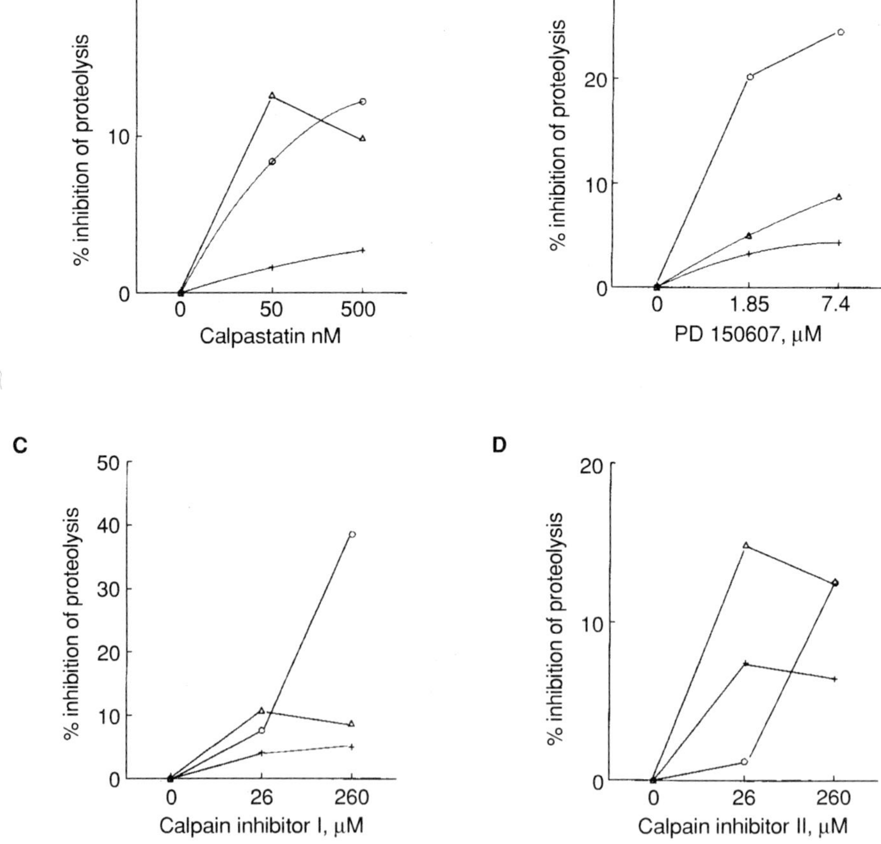

FIGURE 3. Presence of G-actin fragments in PBMC extracts positive for the presence of the 37-kDa 2-5A-BP. Human G-actin (control, lanes 1A and 1B), and cell extracts (lanes 2-5) were analyzed by SDS-PAGE, blotted on membranes before detection with antibodies specific for either the N- (part A) or C-terminal end (part B) of G-actin. The cell extracts analyzed were progressively positive for the presence of the 37-kDa 2-5A-BP from lane 5 to 2, with the percentage of 80-kDa RNase L being, respectively, 98.3, 70.9, 32.5 and 14.8.

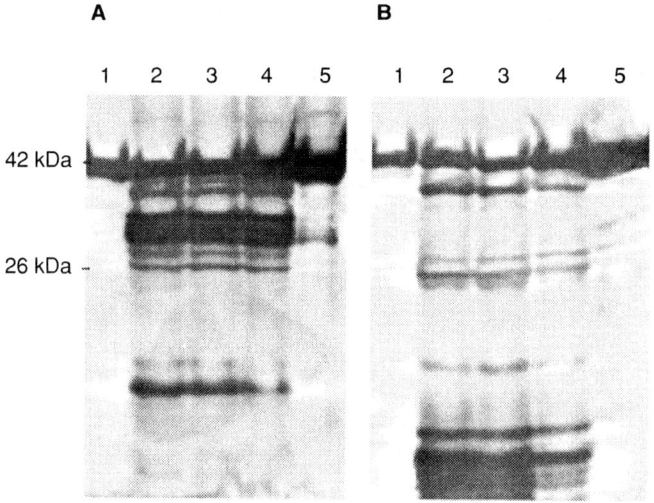

several LMW fragments of G-actin and the preliminary results were likely to indicate that their presence paralleled the presence of the 37-kDa 2-5A-BP. This is already apparent in Figure 3 where the PBMC extracts strongly positive for the presence of the 37-kDa 2-5A-BP show the highest levels of G-actin fragments (lanes 2 and 3) when compared to the less positive samples (lanes 4 and 5). In order to verify further this apparent correlation, we analyzed a significant number of PBMC samples in parallel for the presence of RNase L and G-actin fragments. In this case, we detected the G-actin fragments with the antibody specific for the C-terminal portion of the protein and expressed the results for both proteins as the percentage of the native protein (80-kDa RNase L and 42-kDa G-actin) over total immunoreactive or 2-5A-binding proteins present in the sample, respectively. The results of this correlation study, displayed in Figure 4, show that the percentage of the two native cellular proteins correlated significantly (n = 107; r = 0.707; p < 0.001).

FIGURE 4. Correlation between the percentages of 42-kDa G-actin and 80-kDa RNase L over either total immunoreactive or 2-5A-binding proteins in PBMC extracts (n = 107). Actin was analyzed by immunoblotting using an antibody specific for the C-terminus for detection, and RNase L by SDS-PAGE using a 2-5A radioactive probe for the detection. The correlation (r = 0.707) is highly significant (p < 0.001). The regression line is y = 0.748 x + 18.45.

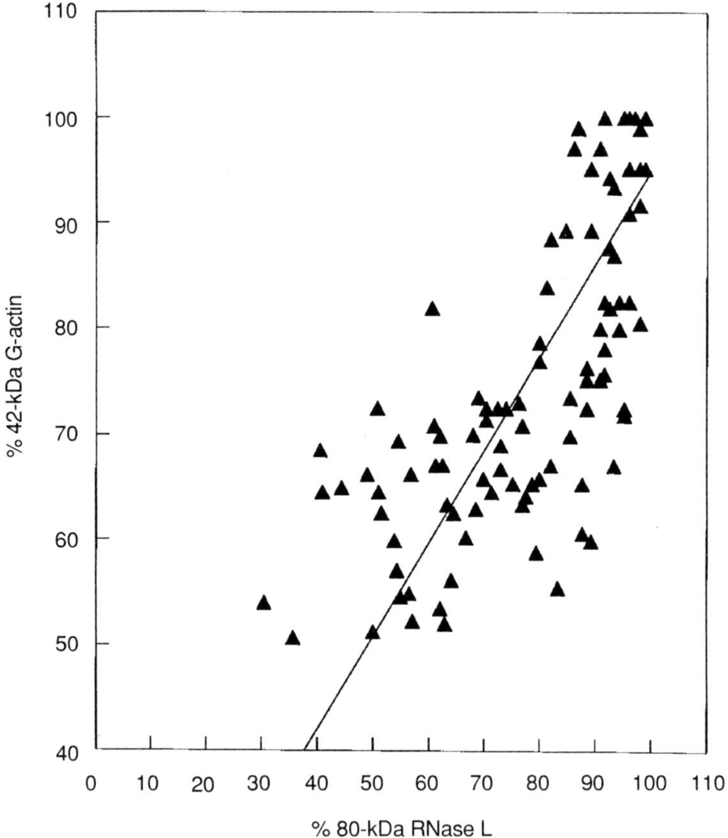

In order to better understand this relationship, we examined the cleavage of G-actin by caspase-3 and calpain in the absence or presence of their inhibitors, respectively (data not shown). Counter to RNase L which is likely to be cleaved by calpain, not the caspase, G-actin was cleaved by both enzymes and the size of the fragments produced matched that of the fragments identified in PBMC.

The Presence of G-Actin Fragments in Serum Reflects the Presence of G-Actin and RNase L Fragments in PBMC

Monomeric G-actin is cleared from the intracellular space as carried by the serum vitamin D-binding protein (Gc component) (16). Previously, it had also been shown that this serum transport protein was also capable of binding G-actin fragments resulting from partial trypsin proteolysis (21). Consequently, this study would have been incomplete if we had not examined serum samples for the possible presence of G-actin fragments (Figure 5). G-actin fragments could not be detected in serum when using the C-terminal antibody (Figure 5B). However, as

FIGURE 5. Actin fragments can be detected by immunoblotting using an antibody specific for the N-terminus of the protein in serum samples matching PBMC samples positive for the presence of the 37-kDa 2-5A-BP. Bovine G-actin (control, lanes 1A and 1B), and serum samples (lanes 2-5) were analyzed by SDS-PAGE and blotted on membranes before detection with antibodies specific for either the N- (part A) or C-terminal end (part B) of G-actin. The serum samples shown in parts A and B matched the PBMC extracts shown in Figure 3 (progressively positive for the presence of the 37-kDa 2-5A-BP in increasing order from lane 5 to 2). Parts C and D present the detection of N-terminal immunoreactive forms of actin on immunoblots of serum samples matching PBMC samples either negative (part C) or positive (part D) for the presence of the 37-kDa 2-5A-BP.

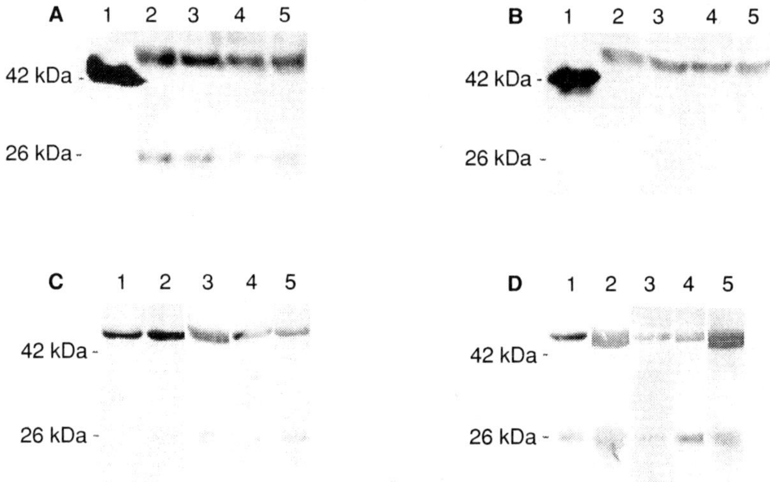

shown in Figure 5A, monomeric G-actin and a 26-kDa fragment were detected when the N-terminal antibody was used. Using the same N-terminal antibody, the fragment was hardly detectable in serum samples matching PBMC samples negative for the presence of the 37-kDa 2-5A-BP (Figure 5C). Counter to that (Figure 5D), the actin fragment was clearly visible in serum samples matching PBMC samples positive for the presence of the 37-kDa 2-5A-BP. In serum, the apparent molecular weight of monomeric G-actin was quite higher than what was observed in the PBMC extracts. This most probably results from the presence of the serum binding protein which, due to its huge affinity (K_A 1.7 $\times$ 10^9 mol^{-1}) for G-actin (22), cannot be detached completely from the complexes even in reduced conditions. We further performed a correlation study (Figure 6) with matching serum-PBMC samples and found a highly significant relationship (r = 0.64; p < 0.001) between the percentage of monomeric G-actin over total immunoreactive actin in either serum or PBMC. In view of the highly significant correlation existing between the presence of monomeric G-actin and RNase L fragments in PBMC (see Figure 4 in text), we calculated the correlation between the percentage of high molecular weight G-actin in serum and the percentage of native 80-kDa 2-5A-binding RNase L in matched PBMC samples (n = 175). As shown in Figure 7, the correlation indicated statistical significance (r = 0.4; p < 0.001). When we applied as a normality threshold for serum actin level, the percentage of the high molecular weight form crossing the normality threshold for the RNase L assay in PBMC (see Figure 7, dotted lines), the respective sensitivity and specificity of the serum actin test were 92.6 and 98.3%.

DISCUSSION

The present study was undertaken to explore the possibility that a proteolytic cleavage of RNase L could be at the origin of the 37-kDa 2-5A-BP present in the PBMC of CFS patients (13,14). This possibility had been previously suggested by several observations, including the separate genetic expression of the LMW enzyme (13). In order to resolve this important issue, we used r-hRNase L labeled with radioactive 2-5A that we incubated progressively with PBMC extracts either positive or negative for the 37-kDa 2-5A-BP. Only the positive extracts generated the fragments in a significant amount during incubation (Figure 1B, lanes 5-10), and the fragment generated matched the size of the fragment observed with the native sample enzyme (Figure 1A). With

FIGURE 6. Correlation between the presence of G-actin fragments in serum and in PBMC. Matching samples (n = 68) were correlated for their content in percent of high molecular weight (MW) G-actin in serum and percent of 42-kDa G-actin in PBMC, respectively. Actin and its fragments were detected by immunoblotting using an antibody specific for the N-terminal end. The regression line is y = 1.3 x − 19. The correlation (r = 0.64) is highly significant (p < 0.001).

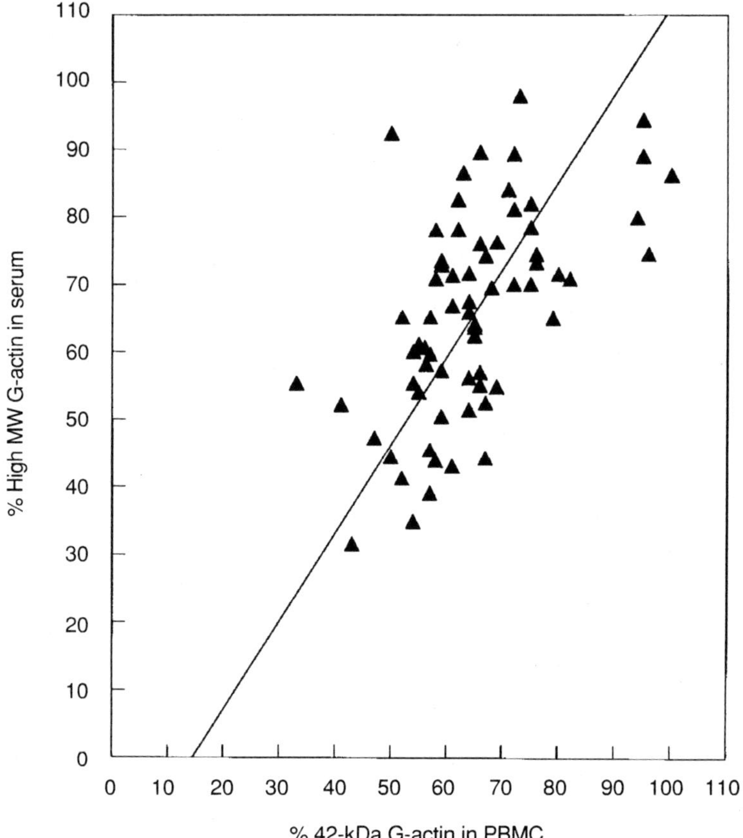

the positive PBMC extracts, the signal of the 80-kDa band decreased progressively with incubation time, as the result of the progressive appearance of the LMW fragment. This progressive decrease of the 80-kDa band with incubation further supports the conclusion that the 37-kDa 2-5A-BP arises by cleavage of the monomeric RNase L. Because the cocktail added during PBMC preparation contained inhibitors

FIGURE 7. Correlation between the presence of G-actin fragments in serum and RNase L fragments in PBMC. Matching samples (n = 175) were correlated for their content in percent of high molecular weight (MW) G-actin in serum and percent of 80-kDa RNase L in PBMC, respectively. Actin was analyzed in serum by immunoblotting using an antibody specific for the N-terminal end and RNase L by SDS-PAGE using a 2-5A radioactive probe for the detection. The regression line is y = 0.843 x + 2.49. The correlation (r = 0.4) is highly significant (p < 0.001). When a threshold for normality is applied for serum actin, corresponding to the threshold of normality for RNase L in PBMC (dotted lines), the sensitivity and specificity of the actin serum test are, respectively, 92.6 and 98.3% of those of the RNase L PBMC assay.

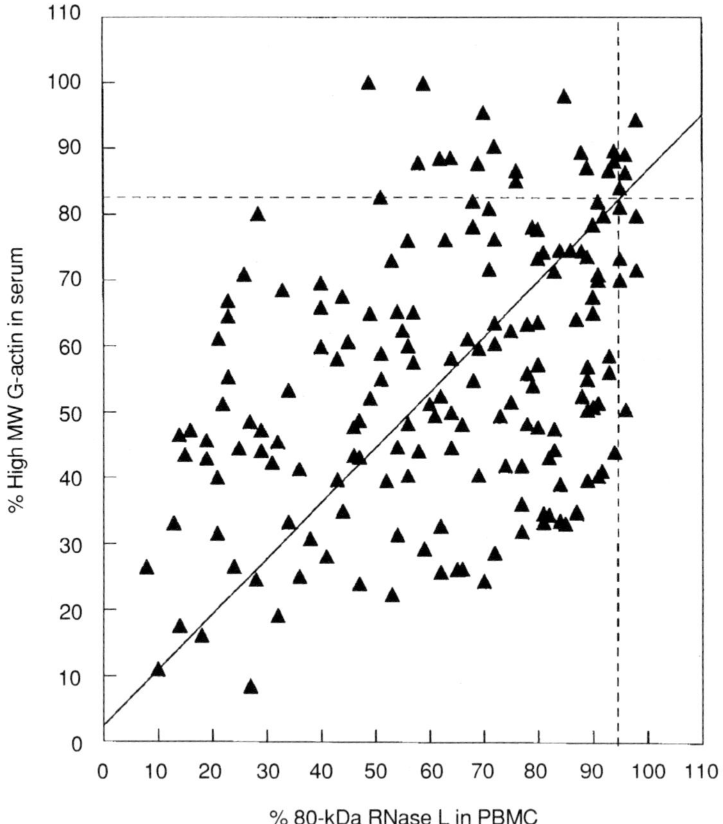

to most protease families, excluding specific inhibitors to the cysteine proteases, we investigated two members of this latter family, namely caspase-3 and calpain, as possible candidates for the proteolytic activity observed. As we demonstrate here (Figure 1C), calpain, but not the caspase, is likely to be involved in the generation of the 37-kDa 2-5A-BP. The specific involvement of calpain in the production of the LMW 2-5A-BP by cell extracts is further exemplified in Figures 1D and 2, which show that the cleavage is partially reduced when calpain had been previously immunoprecipitated (Figure 1D), or when calpain inhibitors are present (Figure 2) during the incubation. However, failure to completely inhibit the cleavage of the 80-kDa enzyme in a 37-kDa fragment in these conditions is likely to indicate that calpain is not the only protease involved in the process.

Calpain is a cysteine protease particularly active during apoptosis (19). Increased proportions apoptotic populations have been previously observed in the PBMC of CFS patients and an increased expression of protein kinase R has been held responsible for this dysfunction (15). However, RNase L itself is capable of inducing apoptosis (23,24), and because of its unregulation in CFS (11), one can probably suggest that the protein plays also a critical role in the increased induction of apoptosis in CFS PBMC. Among the cellular substrates of calpain, G-actin has been probably one of the most studied (25,26). The protein has also been shown to be cleaved by caspase-3 *in vitro* (27) whilst it has been suggested that the protein could withstand cleavage by this enzyme *in vivo* (28). Nevertheless, we show here that G-actin fragments are present in the PBMC containing the 37-kDa 2-5A-BP (Figure 3) and that the percentages of the high molecular weight forms of both proteins in PBMC extracts correlate significantly (Figure 4). Our experiments with purified caspase-3 and calpain confirm that unlike RNase L, which is likely to be cleaved by calpain only, both enzymes are able to cleave G-actin *in vitro,* as previously reported (25-27). Because G-actin plays a critical role in antigen presentation and T-cell signaling (reviewed in 29), an increased G-actin cleavage in the mononuclear cells of CFS patients might partly explain the numerous immunological disorders from which they suffer (5-7).

Finally, we show that a G-actin fragment is retrieved only in serum samples matching PBMC samples positive for the presence of the 37-kDa 2-5A-BP (Figure 5). The percentage of high molecular weight actin in serum further correlates with the percentage of 42-kDa G-actin in PBMC (Figure 6). This is consistent with the fact that monomeric G-actin and at least one of its low molecular weight fragments are cleared from damaged cells by serum transport bound with high affinity by the vitamin D-binding protein (16,21,22). This serum fragment could be detected only when an antibody specific for the N-terminal sequence of G-actin was used, suggesting that the fragment detected lacks the C-terminal part of the protein. We also show in this report that the presence of the G-actin fragment in serum correlates significantly with the presence of the 37-kDa 2-5A-BP in PBMC (Figure 7).

CFS is an illness which was devoid of any *in vitro* diagnostic test (30) until very recently, when the detection of the 37-kDa 2-5A-BP in PBMC was suggested as a potential marker for the syndrome (14). At the one hand, the test requires a quite high quantity of blood, which might be inconvenient to the patient, and at the other hand the assay requires a high technical expertise to be performed and is consequently expensive. An assay detecting the presence of the G-actin fragment in serum may thus be useful as a screening test for CFS and would reduce the inconvenience and cost to both the patient and healthcare system. However, similar observations of the presence of G-actin fragments in serum have been reported previously in severe liver necrosis (31,32) and the test might consequently lack clinical specificity for CFS. However, when we applied as a normality threshold for serum actin the percentage value of the high molecular weight form crossing the normality threshold for the 37-kDa 2-5A-BP assay in PBMC (14), the sensitivity and specificity of the serum actin test were respectively 92.6 and 98.3% of those of the 37-kDa 2-5A-BP PBMC test. Consequently, the serum actin test is likely to provide a biological information which is very close to that provided by the 37-kDa 2-5A-BP assay in PBMC. As with any clinical assay used as a screening test, a positive result should be confirmed by the PBMC assay for 37-kDa 2-5A-BP and confronted to all clinical data available before making a definitive medical diagnosis of CFS.

REFERENCES

1. Williams BRG, Golgher RR, Brown RE, et al. Natural occurrence of 2-5A in interferon-treated EMC virus-infected L cells. *Nature* 1979; *282*: 582-586.

2. Maitra RK, Li G, Xiao W, et al. Catalytic cleavage of an RNA target by 2-5A antisense and RNase L. *J. Biol. Chem.* 1995; *270*: 15071-15075.

3. Dong B, Silverman RH. 2-5A-dependent RNase molecules dimerize during activation by 2-5A. *J. Biol. Chem.* 1995; *270*: 4133-4137.

4. Wreschner DH, McCauley JW, Skehel JJ, et al. Interferon action–Sequence specificity of the $ppp(A2'p)_nA$-dependent ribonuclease. *Nature* 1981; *289*: 414-417.

5. Komaroff AL, Buchwald DS. Chronic fatigue syndrome: An update. *Annu. Rev. Med.* 1998; *49*: 1-13.

6. Konstantinov K, Von Miekecz A, Buchwald D, et al. Autoantibodies to nuclear envelope antigens in chronic fatigue syndrome. *J. Clin. Invest.* 1996; *98*: 1888-1896.

7. Landay AL, Jessop C, Lennette ET, et al. Chronic fatigue syndrome: Condition associated with immune activation. *Lancet* 1991; *338*: 707-712.

8. Strauss SE, Komaroff AL, Wedner HJ. Chronic fatigue syndrome: Point and counterpoint. *J. Infect. Dis.* 1994; *170*: 1-6.

9. Swanink CMA., Vercoulen JHMM., Bleijenberg G., et al. Chronic fatigue syndrome: A clinical and laboratory study with a well matched control group. *J. Intern. Med.* 1995; *237*: 499-506.

10. Visser J, Blauw B, Hinloopen B, et al. CD4 T Lymphocytes from patients with chronic fatigue syndrome have decreased interferon-γ production and increased sensitivity to dexamethasone. *J. Infect. Dis.* 1998; *177*: 451-454.

11. Suhadolnik RJ, Reichenbach NL, Hitzges P, et al. Upregulation of the 2-5A synthetase/RNase L antiviral pathway associated with chronic fatigue syndrome. *Clin. Infect. Dis.* 1994; *18*: S96-S104.

12. Suhadolnik RJ, Reichenbach NL, Hitzges P, et al. Changes in the 2-5A synthetase/RNase L antiviral pathway in a controlled clinical trial with Poly(I)-Poly($C_{12}U$) in chronic fatigue syndrome. *In Vivo* 1994; *8*: 599-604.

13. Suhadolnik RJ, Peterson DL, O'Brien K, et al. Biochemical evidence for a novel low molecular weight 2-5A-dependent RNase L in chronic fatigue syndrome. *J. Interferon Cytokine Res.* 1997; *17*: 377-385.

14. De Meirleir K, Bisbal C, Campine I, et al. A 37 kDa 2-5A binding protein as a potential biochemical marker for chronic fatigue syndrome. *Am. J. Med.* 2000; *108*: 99-105.

15. Vojdani A, Ghoneum M, Choppa PC, et al. Elevated apoptotic cell population in patients with chronic fatigue syndrome: The pivotal role of protein kinase RNA. *J. Intern. Med.* 1997; *242*: 465-478.

16. Coue M, Constans J, Olomucki A. Effects of serum vitamin-D-binding protein on actin in the presence of plasma gelsolin. *Eur. J. Biochem.* 1986; *160*: 273-277.

17. Zhou A, Hassel BA, Silverman RH. Expression cloning of 2-5A-dependent RNAase: A uniquely regulated mediator of interferon action. *Cell* 1993; *72*: 753-765.

18. Earnshaw WC, Martins LM, Kaufmann SH. Mammalian caspases: Structure, activation, substrates, and functions during apoptosis. *Annu. Rev. Biochem.* 1999; *68*: 383-424.

19. Saido TC, Sorimachi H, Suzuki K. Calpain: New perspectives in molecular diversity and physiological-pathological involvement. *FASEB J.* 1994; *8*: 814-822.

20. Mashima T, Naito M, Tsuruo T. Caspase-mediated cleavage of cytoskeletal actin plays a positive role in the process of morphological apoptosis. *Oncogene* 1999; *18*: 2423-2430.

21. Goldschmidt-Clermont P, Allen RC, Nel AE, et al. Gc (vitamin D-binding protein) binds the 33.5 K tryptic fragment of actin. *Life Sci.* 1986; *38*: 735-742.

22. Mc Leod JF, Kowalski MA, Haddad JG. Jr Interactions among serum vitamin D binding protein, monomeric actin, profilin and profilactin. *J. Biol. Chem.* 1989; *264*: 1260-1267.

23. Diaz-Guerra M, Rivas C, Esteban M. Activation of the IFN-inducible enzyme RNase L causes apoptosis of animal cells. *Virology* 1997; *236*: 354-363.

24. Castelli JC, Hassel BA, Wood KA, et al. A study of the interferon antiviral mechanism: Apoptosis activation by the 2-5A system. *J. Exp. Med.* 1997; *186*: 967-972.

25. Villa G, Henzel WJ, Sensenbrenner M, et al. Calpain inhibitors, but not caspase inhibitors, prevent actin proteolysis and DNA fragmentation during apoptosis. *J. Cell Sci.* 1998; *111*: 713-722.

26. Brown SB, Bailey K, Savill J. Actin is cleaved during constitutive apoptosis. *Biochem. J.* 1997; *323*: 233-237.

27. Mashima T, Naito M, Noguchi K, et al. Actin cleavage by CPP32/apopain during the development of apoptosis. *Oncogene* 1997; *14*: 1007-1012.

28. Song Q, Wei T, Lees-Miller S, et al. Resistance of actin to cleavage during apoptosis. *Proc. Nat. Acad. Sci. USA* 1997; *94*: 157-162.

29. Dustin ML, Cooper JA. The immunological synapse and the actin cytoskeleton: Molecular hardware for T cell signaling. *Nature Immunol.* 2000; *1*: 23-29.

30. Komaroff AL. The biology of chronic fatigue syndrome. *Am. J. Med.* 2000; *108*: 169-171.

31. Goldschmidt-Clermont PJ, Galbraith RM, Emerson DL, et al. Accurate quantitation of native Gc in serum and estimation of endogenous Gc:G-actin complexes by rocket immunoelectrophoresis. *Clin. Chim. Acta* 1985; *148*: 173-183.

32. Young WO, Goldschmidt-Clermont P, Emerson DL, et al. Correlation between extent of liver damage in fulminant hepatic necrosis and complexing of circulating group-specific component (vitamin D-binding protein). *J. Lab. Clin. Med.* 1987; *110*: 83-90.

Interactions Between Rnase L Ankyrin-Like Domain and ABC Transporters as a Possible Origin for Pain, Ion Transport, CNS and Immune Disorders of Chronic Fatigue Immune Dysfunction Syndrome

Patrick Englebienne, PhD
C. Vincent Herst, PhD
Karen De Smet, PhD
Anne D'Haese, MS
Kenny De Meirleir, MD, PhD

SUMMARY. Low molecular weight (LMW) ribonuclease L (RNase L) forms have been identified in peripheral blood mononuclear cells (PBMC) of patients with chronic fatigue immune dysfunction syndrome (CFIDS). Data from our laboratory indicate that these LMW RNase L proteins are

---

Patrick Englebienne is affiliated with the Université Libre de Bruxelles (Brugmann Hospital) and is Consultant, RED Laboratories, Brussels, Belgium.

C. Vincent Herst, Karen De Smet and Anne D'Haese are affiliated with the R&D Department of RED Laboratories, Brussels, Belgium.

Kenny De Meirleir is affiliated with the Vrije Universiteit Brussel, Brussels, Belgium.

Address correspondence to: Patrick Englebienne, PhD, RED Laboratories, N.V., Pontbeek 61, B-1731 Zellik, Belgium (E-mail: penglebienne@redlabs.be).

[Haworth co-indexing entry note]: "Interactions Between Rnase L Ankyrin-Like Domain and ABC Transporters as a Possible Origin for Pain, Ion Transport, CNS and Immune Disorders of Chronic Fatigue Immune Dysfunction Syndrome." Englebienne, Patrick et al. Co-published simultaneously in *Journal of Chronic Fatigue Syndrome* (The Haworth Medical Press, an imprint of The Haworth Press, Inc.) Vol. 8, No. 3/4, 2001, pp. 83-102; and: *Innovations in Chronic Fatigue Syndrome Research and Clinical Practice* (ed: Roberto Patarca-Montero) The Haworth Medical Press, an imprint of The Haworth Press, Inc., 2001, pp. 83-102. Single or multiple copies of this article are available for a fee from The Haworth Document Delivery Service [1-800-342-9678, 9:00 a.m. - 5:00 p.m. (EST). E-mail address: getinfo@haworthpressinc.com].

produced by proteolytic cleavage of the native monomeric enzyme and we have identified calpain as one of the possible proteases involved. Using human recombinant RNase L (r-hRNase L) His-tagged at the N-terminus, we show here at the one hand that both calpain and PBMC extracts from CFIDS patients cleave the protein in fragments of identical sizes containing ankyrin-like repeat sequences. At the other hand, the activity of RNase L is modulated by its interaction with a specific inhibitor (RLI), a member of the ATP binding cassette (ABC) superfamily. RLI interacts with the ankyrin domain of RNase L, which results in a blockade of the 2′,5′-oligoadenylate (2-5A)-binding site of the enzyme. We show that RLI contains a small ankyrin-interacting peptide cluster through which it interacts with the first two β-hairpin coils of the RNase L ankyrin domain. A similarity search performed at the NCBI using RLI aminoacid sequence as the entry allowed to identify several other ABC transporter proteins sharing significant identities with RLI, including the ankyrin-interacting peptide. Taken together, these results show that upon pathological cleavage of RNase L, fragments containing the ankyrin domain are released, which could be capable of interacting with selected members of the human ABC superfamily, preventing their interaction with the normal cognate ankyrin protein and hence impairing their proper cellular function. This interaction constitutes a common physiological mechanism explaining numerous and currently unexplained symptoms experienced by patients with CFIDS, which are otherwise totally unrelated. *[Article copies available for a fee from The Haworth Document Delivery Service: 1-800-342-9678. E-mail address: <getinfo@haworthpressinc. com> Website: <http://www.HaworthPress.com> © 2001 by The Haworth Press, Inc. All rights reserved.]*

KEYWORDS. RNase L, ankyrin-like domain, ABC transporters, CFIDS, CFS, protein interactions, RLI, sequence homology, 3D-models, integral membrane components, cytoskeleton

INTRODUCTION

Ribonuclease L (RNase L) is an endonuclease central to the 2-5A antiviral pathway (1). Upon binding small 2′,5′-oligoadenylates (2-5A) produced from ATP by the 2-5A synthetase activated by interferon and double stranded RNA (ds-RNA), the enzyme homodimerizes. Homodimerization confers the catalytic activity to the protein which cleaves single stranded RNA (ss-RNA) (2). The catalytic activity of RNase L is regulated through interaction with the specific RNase L inhibitor (RLI)

(3,4), which impairs 2-5A-binding to, homodimerization and hence catalytic activation of the monomeric enzyme. The 2-5A-binding site of RNase L is located in the ankyrin-like N-terminal domain of the enzyme which is involved in the interaction with RLI (5).

In chronic fatigue immune dysfunction syndrome (CFIDS), the 2-5A pathway is dysregulated and peripheral blood mononuclear cell (PBMC) extracts are characterized by an unregulated RNase L activity, a down-regulated RLI, and the presence of low molecular weight (LMW) forms of RNase L, including a 37-kDa 2-5A-binding protein (37-kDa RNase L) (6-8). Besides cellular and humoral immunity dysfunctions (9), patients suffering from CFIDS present also many symptoms, including pain, which are likely to reflect dysregulations in both ion and amino acid transport (10,11). The involvement of ion channel dysfunction in CFIDS has already been proposed, based on clinical observation (10,12), as a rationale for some of the symptoms observed in the illness.

A recent study (13) classifies RLI as a member of the ATP binding cassette (ABC) superfamily of ion membrane transporters. We show here that RLI sequence shares strong homologies with other members of the superfamily, which include a small peptide ankyrin-binding motif analogous to the tetra- or pentapeptide through which, both the Na^+,K^+-ATPase and erythroid anion exchanger AE1 interact with the erythrocyte ankyrin (14,15). We report also that the PBMC of CFIDS patients contain a proteolytic activity which cleaves RNase L in fragments containing the ankyrin-like domain. Ankyrins are heterobifunctional proteins which play fundamental roles in linking the cytoplasmic domain of integral membrane proteins to the cytoskeleton (14,15). Our results strongly suggest that the ankyrin fragments released from RNase L in cells of CFIDS patients are capable of interacting with members of the ABC superfamily homologous to RLI. This could preclude their interaction with the normal cognate ankyrin protein and result in a dysregulation of their normal ion channeling function.

MATERIALS AND METHODS

Study Subjects and Samples

Study subjects were individuals selected from a medical practice at the University of Brussels for the 37-kDa RNase L analysis in PBMC as previously described (8). PBMC samples remaining after the routine assays had been performed were used in this study.

Peripheral Blood Mononuclear Cells (PBMC) Extracts

PBMC were separated from heparinized blood by Ficoll-Hypaque density gradient centrifugation within four hours of blood draw as previously described (6). The PBMCs were then stored at $-70°C$ until cytoplasmic extracts could be made. Cytoplasmic extracts were prepared in the presence of the protease inhibitors aprotinin, leupeptin, pefabloc-SC and EDTA (Roche Biochemicals, Mannheim, Germany). Total proteins were measured in the cell extracts using a modified Bradford assay method (Bio-Rad Laboratories, Hercules, CA) according to the manufacturer's procedure. The cytoplasmic extracts were normalized for total protein content in each experiment.

Production of Recombinant Human RNase L
(r-hRNase L) Protein

r-hRNaseL was cloned, and expressed in baculovirus transfected Sf21 insect cells by ATG Laboratories (Eden Prairie, MN). An His6-tag was inserted at the aminoterminus of the protein which was purified to 90-95% homogeneity by metal chelate chromatography on Ni-Nitrilotriacetic acid-agarose. A monoclonal antibody raised against tetrahistidine (Qiagen, Venlo, The Netherlands) specifically recognizes a single band in the purified protein solution with an apparent molecular weight of 84-kDa by SDS-PAGE.

In Vitro Cleavage of r-hRNase L by PBMC
Extracts and Calpain

r-hRNase L (1.3 µg) was incubated at 37°C during 30 minutes with either 200 µg of PBMC proteins or 0.42 unit neutral calpain (m-calpain, Sigma, St. Louis, MO), respectively. Proteins were then resolved by 10% SDS-PAGE. The separated proteins were then transferred to a 0.2 µm PVDF membrane (Bio-Rad Laboratories, Hercules, CA) using a semi-dry transfer system (Amersham-Pharmacia Biotech, Amersham, UK). Transfer was performed at an average current of 0.8 mA per cm² for two hours. After transfer was complete, the membrane was allowed to dry thoroughly at room temperature for at least one hour. The membrane was then wet with a minimum volume of 100% methanol, subsequently replaced by a solution of 5% (w:v) non-fat dry milk in phosphate-buffered saline, pH 7.4 containing 0.1% (v:v) Tween 20 (PBS-Tween) as blocking buffer and the membrane was incubated for one hour with gentle shaking. The blocking buffer was discarded and fresh blocking buffer containing the primary antibody (1:300, v:v dilution in PBS of horseradish peroxidase-labeled anti-His monoclonal antibody from Sigma, St. Louis, MO). The membrane was allowed to react with the antibody for one hour with gentle shaking. The primary antibody solution was then discarded and the membrane was washed three times with 25 ml PBS-Tween. Color development was then performed using the Opti4-CN® kit from Bio-Rad Laboratories (Hercules, CA).

Molecular Modelling

The three-dimensional (3D)-molecular models of RNase L and RLI were constructed by usual bioinformatic procedures. The protein data bank (Pdb) was searched using the respective amino acid sequences of RNase L and RLI using FASTA (16) and BLAST (17) programs at either the European Bioinformatics Institute (Hinxton, UK), or at the National Center for Biotechnology Information (NCBI, Bethesda, MD). The sequences of the proteins to be modelled where then threaded on the matching 3D structures from the Pdb (18,19) using the Swiss-model facility at the Expasy server (http://www.expasy.ch). The models were further assembled and displayed using WebLab Viewer 3.7 (Molecular Simulations, Inc.) and were subjected to Ramachandran's analysis for accuracy (20).

Sequence Similarity Search

The aminoacid sequence of RLI was used as the entry to search the Genbank at NCBI for sequence similarities using the BLAST program (17). Sequence aligments were performed using Clustal W as the program (21).

RESULTS

Production of 37-kDa RNase L in PBMC of CFIDS Patients Is Accompanied by the Release of N-Terminal Ankyrin Fragments

The human monomeric RNase L is a polypeptide made of 741 aminoacids with a molecular mass of 83-kDa (22). The protein sequence contains several interesting molecular features. From the N-terminal end, the first 330 amino acid residues are structured as nine ankyrin repeat motifs. Figure 1 shows the homology between the aligned ankyrin repeat sequences of RNase L and the ankyrin motif consensus (23). The identities with the consensus motif lie between 54 and 77%. This ankyrin-like domain includes the 2-5A-binding site of the protein partly made of two conserved P-loop motifs (GKT) (residues 239-241 and 273-275) present at the same relative positions of the seventh and eighth ankyrin repeats (boxed in Figure 1). Farther in the sequence, the protein is characterized by a protein kinase-like domain

FIGURE 1. Sequence aligment of the nine ankyrin repeats of human RNase L with the ankyrin consensus. Identities are in bold and underlined. Gaps are represented by dashes and X represents any aminoacid. The two P-loops are boxed.

Ankyrin-Repeat Consensus:

```
XGXTP-------------LHXAAXXXX---XXXVXXLLXX-GAXXXXXXDX

XGXTP-------------AHXAAXXXX---XXXVXXLLXX-GAXXXXXXNX
```

RNase L Sequence:

```
 11  EGPTSSSGRRAAVEDNHLLIKAVQNED---VDLVQQLLEG-GANVNFQEEE

 58  GGWTP-----------LHNAVQMSR---EDIVELLLRH-GADPVLRKK-

 91  NGATP-----------FILAAIAGS---VKLLKLFLSK-GADVNECDF-

124  YGFTA-----------FMEAAVYGK---VKALKFLYKR-GANVNLRRKT

167  GGATA-----------LMDAAEKGH---VEVLKILLDEMGADVNACDN-

201  MGRNA-----------LIHALLSSDDSDVEAITHLLLDHGADVNVRGER

238  RGKTP-----------LILAVEKKH---LGLVQRLLEQEHIEINDTDSD

272  DGKTA-----------LLLAVELKL----KKIAELLCKRGASTDCGDL-

301  CGDLV-------------MTARRNYD---HSLVKVLLSH-GAKEDFHPPA
```

which includes a cys-rich sequence (residues 390-490) reminiscent of the finger-like structure of proteins pertaining to the thyroid/steroid-receptor superfamily (24). Finally, the catalytic site is located at the C-terminus (5).

Experimental evidence from our laboratory (data not shown) indicates that the 37-kDa 2-5A-binding protein present in the PBMC extracts of patients with CFIDS (6-8) is produced by proteolytic cleavage of the monomeric enzyme. Among the cellular proteolytic enzymes possibly involved, calpain has been identified as capable of generating i.a. the 37-kDa protein. Therefore, we wanted to see if besides the fragments containing the 2-5A-binding site of the enzyme, calpain and PBMC extracts were also able of generating fragments containing the N-terminus of RNase L and its associated ankyrin-like repeats. To this aim, we used r-hRNase L of which the N-terminus was tagged with a hexaHis motif. We incubated the r-hRNase L with either recombinant calpain or PBMC extracts previously analyzed and found them to be positive for the presence of the 37-kDa protein (8). We detected the fragments generated from the r-hRNase L by immunoblotting, using a monoclonal anti-His antibody. The fragments detected by this procedure contain the ankyrin-like N-terminus of RNase L. As shown in Figure 2A, calpain was able to generate N-terminal fragments with apparent molecular weights identical to those fragments generated by the PBMC extracts. Interestingly, the 37-kDa 2-5A-binding protein was not detected by this procedure, which is likely to indicate that this protein is devoid of the N-terminus sequence of native RNase L. It is also worth to notice, as shown in Figure 2A (lane 2) and B, that some of the fragments generated have MW between 15 and 25-kDa, which corresponds to fragments containing the first 4-6 ankyrin repeats of RNase L, excluding the 2-5A-binding site (see Figure 1).

RLI Is a Member of the ATP-Binding Cassette Superfamily

RLI is a 599-amino acid long protein which forms heterodimers with monomeric RNase L (3,4). From the N-terminus, the protein sequence is characterized by a domain containing the ferredoxin iron-binding region signature ($CX_2CX_2CX_3$[PEG], residues 55-66). Recently (13), RLI has been classified in the superfamily of the human ABC transport proteins. Like many members of this superfamily, the amino acid sequence of RLI contains two P-loop consensus motifs (GX_4GK[TS], residues 110-117 and 379-386, respectively), as well as twice the consensus ABC signature pattern (LSGGELQRFACA, residues 217-228 and

FIGURE 2. Calpain and the proteolytic activity of PBMC extracts from CFIDS patients are capable of generating similar RNase L fragments containing the N-terminal ankyrin-repeats of the native enzyme. r-hRNase L containing a His-tag on the N-terminus was incubated with either calpain or patient PBMC extracts. The fragments generated by proteolysis were separated by PAGE and detected by immunoblotting using an anti-His antibody. Part A: Comparison between fragments generated, respectively, from r-hRNase L (lane 1) by a patient extract (lane 2) and calpain (lane 3). Part B: Formation of LMW ankyrin fragments by PBMC extracts containing different levels of the 37-kDa 2-5A-binding protein (as expressed by the 37-kDa/80-kDa ratio), respectively, 2.5 (lane 1), 8.7 (lane 2), and 30.3 (lane 3). Arrows identify fragments of identical sizes.

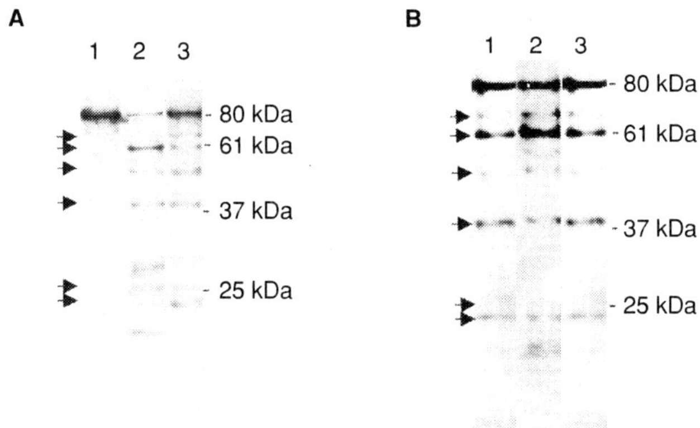

LSGGELQRVRLR, residues 462-473, respectively) (25). Because of this new classification, we made a sequence similarity search at the NCBI which delivered significant homologies with several members of the superfamily. These are summarized in Figure 3. Among the homologies observed, many relate to human multidrug resistance transporters (MDR/TAP subfamily, namely the antigen peptide transporter [TAP1], MDR3, ABC7) and their associated proteins (MRP/CFTR subfamily, namely MRP6, MRP3, the cystic fibrosis transmembrane receptor [CFTR], and the sulfonylurea receptor [SUR1]) (13). Besides these, RLI sequence is also strongly homologous with respectively those of ABC3 which plays a major role in the engulfment of apoptotic cells by macrophages (26), ABC8 (white protein homolog, 27), and retinal-specific ABC transporter (ABCR or Rim protein, 28).

The parts of the sequences of these ABC transporters matching with RLI sequence contain both the two P-loop motifs along with the ABC transporter superfamily consensus pattern.

FIGURE 3. Schematic representation of sequence homologies between human RLI and ABC transporters. Homology levels are: 100%, black; >95%, hatched; 50-55%, dots; 45-50%, grey; 40-45%, crossed; 35-40%, white. The starting and ending residue numbers of the compared sequences matching that of RLI are indicated at left and right of the boxes.

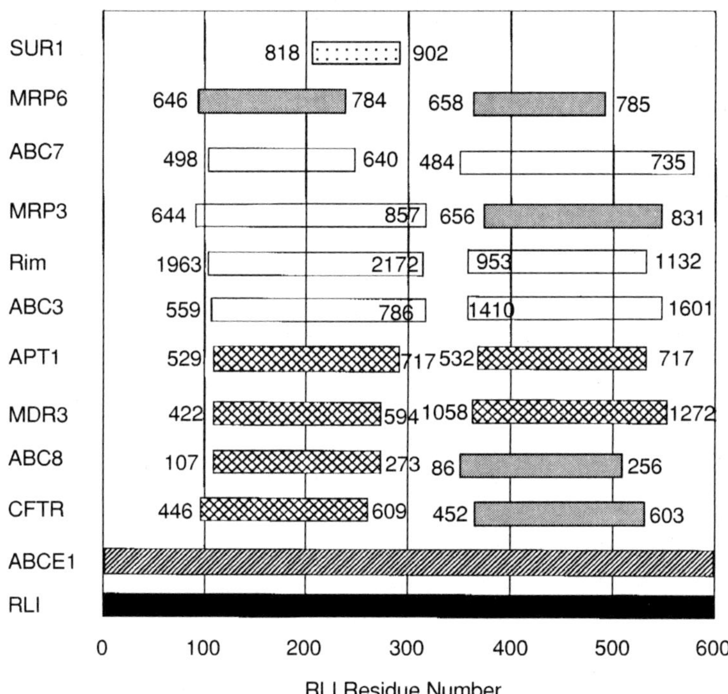

RNase L-RLI Interactions

In order to better understand the interaction of RNase L and RLI, we made 3D models of both proteins. These models were tested for accuracy by being submitted to Ramachandran's analysis (20). The results were 93 and 98% accuracy, respectively, for RNase L and RLI models. It had been shown earlier (3,4) that RLI interacts with the ankyrin domain of RNase L and it was suggested (4) that the ferredoxin iron-binding signature present in the sequence of RLI could be involved in the formation of heterodimers with RNase L. So far however, the ankyrin-binding motif of RLI has not been identified. As we show above, RLI is also an ion transporter of the ABC superfamily. Thus, as other ion channel proteins, RLI could be suspected of interacting with ankyrin proteins through a specific signature sequence (29). Thus, we concurrently analyzed RLI sequence for the presence of possible ankyrin-interacting peptides and we identified a tetrapeptide (AIIK, residues 166-169) strongly analogous to the tetra- or pentapeptide clusters (ALLK and ALLLK, respectively) which have been identified as the ankyrin-binding motifs of respectively the Na^+,K^+-ATPase (14) and erythroid anion exchanger (15). The only difference is a conservative replacement of leucines by isoleucines. This peptide motif could interact by making hydrophobic as well as ionic contacts with residues in the β-hairpin tips of ankyrin proteins. In order to verify the feasibility of this possible interaction, we tethered the respective interacting structures on our model proteins. As shown on Figure 4, the proposed interaction was applied successfully. The binding of RLI to the ankyrin domain of RNase L brings parts of RLI structure very close to the 2-5A-binding site of the enzyme (yellow surface, Figure 4), inducing steric hindrance that could account for the loss of 2-5A-binding activity in the heterodimeric complex (3,4). Moreover, the interaction makes the ferredoxin iron-binding cluster loop of RLI (colored green on Figure 4) to protrude and line-up with the cysteine-rich domain of RNase L. The interaction between the tetrapeptide and the ankyrin domain of RNase L is further illustrated in Figure 5. Hydrophobic contacts are established in the first ankyrin loop between A(166)-F(53) and I(167)-W(60) and in the second ankyrin loops between I(168)-A(93). An ionic contact is finally established between the RLI lysine (169) and threonine (94) of RNase L.

The Ankyrin Fragments Released by RNase L Cleavage Are Able to Interact with the ABC Transporters Homologous to RLI

As we have shown above, RLI sequence is homologous to several ABC transporter proteins and in the PBMC of CFIDS patients, RNase L is cleaved and releases several fragments containing the ankyrin domain. Our 3D-modelling of the RNase L-RLI interaction indicates that the ankyrin domain of the enzyme probably interacts with a peptide motif analogous to that responsible for the interaction of other ion-channel proteins with ankyrins (14,15). It was thus also possible that these

FIGURE 4. Three dimensional model of RNase L (depicted as vdw surface colored according to electric potential) interacting with RLI (depicted in solid ribbon colored according to the secondary structure). RLI binds to the first ankyrin β-hairpin loops of RNase L ankyrin domain through the AIIK tetrapeptide ankyrin-binding motif and blocks the 2-5A-binding site of the enzyme by steric hindrance (yellow surfaces). The interaction further lines the ferredoxin iron-binding cluster of RLI (green) with the cysteine-rich domain of RNase L (left hand part) and competes with cognate enzyme monomers for dimerization.

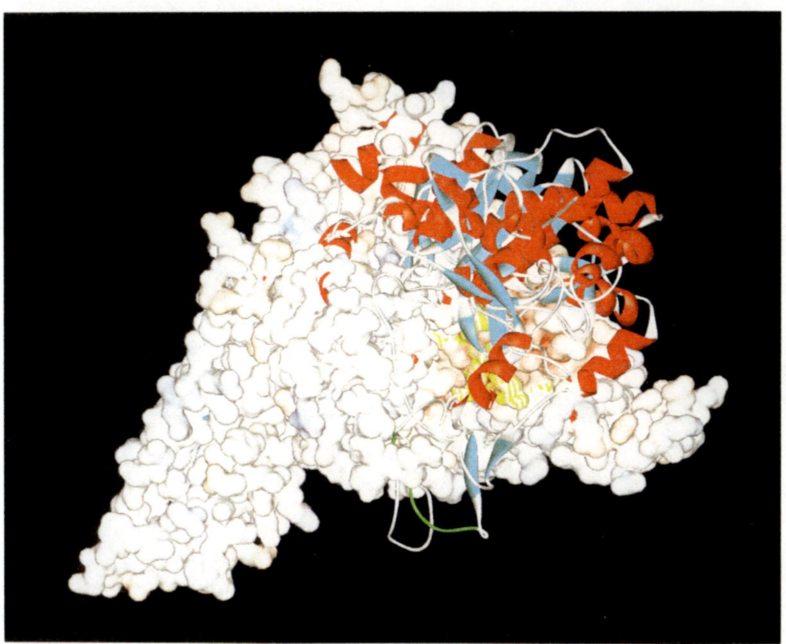

ankyrin fragments released from RNase L were also capable of interaction with the ABC transporters sharing strong homologies with RLI. In order to verify this possibility, we analyzed the sequence of the ABC transporters homologous to RLI for the possible presence of the tetra- or pentapeptide signature which allows RLI along with the Na⁺,K⁺-ATPase and AE1 ion exchangers to interact with ankyrins. As shown in Figure 6, all the ABC transporters considered contain the consensus tetra- or pentapeptide signature, the leucines and isoleucines being alterned and in some cases the terminal lysine being conservatively replaced by an arginine (ABC8 and MDR3) or a glutamine (SUR1).

FIGURE 5. Interaction between RLI tetrapeptide (tube representation) and the two first loops of the ankyrin domain (ribbon) of RNase L. The hydrophobic contacts in the first loop are A(166)-F(53) and I(167)-W(60) and in the second loop I(168)-A(93). A final ionic contact between K(169) of RLI and T(94) in the second ankyrin hairpin loop of RNase L secures the interaction. The respective aminoacids of RLI are labeled in yellow and those of RNase L in green. The surfaces shown correspond to the van der Waals radii.

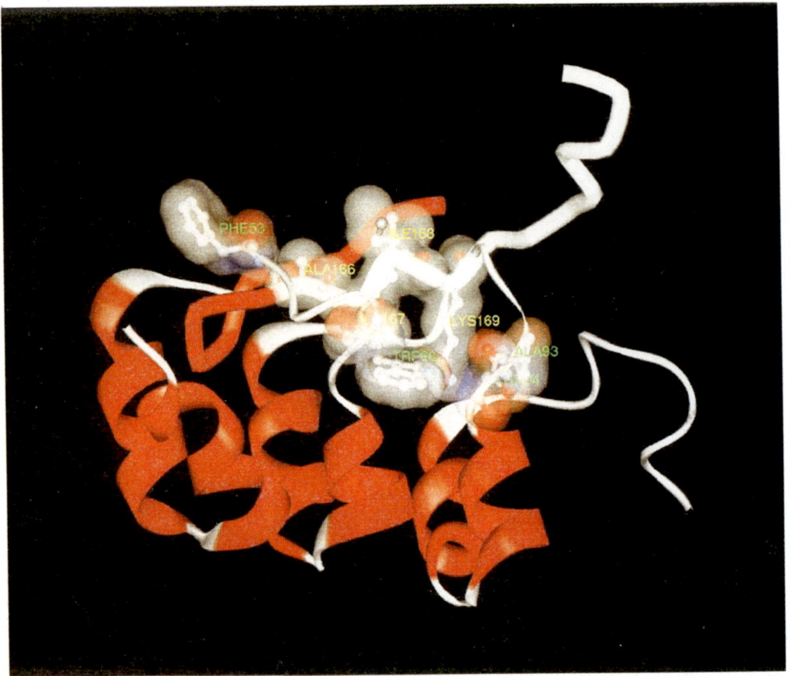

DISCUSSION

The aminoacid sequence of RNase L contains nine ankyrin repeat units (Figure 1) which include the two P-loops associated with the 2-5A-binding site of the protein. RNase L ankyrin repeats interact with the enzyme natural inhibitor RLI (3) and it has been demonstrated (4) that the formation of RLI-RNase L complexes prevents any 2-5A binding to the enzyme, a prerequisite for its homodimerization and catalytic activity attainment (2). By 3D-modelling we show here that this interaction can occur with a tetrapeptide cluster present in RLI sequence which is analogous to the ankyrin-interacting motif of erythrocyte membrane

FIGURE 6. Sequence alignment of RLI and homologous ABC plasma membrane transporter proteins with the tetra- or pentapeptide ankyrin-interacting consensus cluster of Na$^+$, K$^+$-ATPase and AE1. Identities are in bold and conservative replacements are boxed.

Consensus:

AE1	155	RALLLKH
Na$^+$, K$^+$-ATPase	465	SALL-KC

ABC members:

SUR1	363	LALLL[Q]R
MRP6	867	PALL[I]KD
ABC7	621	RA[I]L-KD
MRP3	1438	RALLRKS
Rim	1355	QALLVKR
ABC3	1380	PL[II]-KE
TAP1	655	RAL[I]RKP
MDR3	155	HA[I]L-[R]Q
ABC8	631	EA[I]L-[R]E
CFTR	325	YAL[I]-KG
ABC1	165	KA[II]-KP
RLI	165	KA[II]-KP

ion exchangers. This interaction (Figure 4) brings parts of the RLI structure close to the 2-5A-binding site of RNase L, inducing a steric hindrance preventing any binding of the oligoadenylates. The interaction further makes the ferredoxin iron-binding cluster of RLI to protrude and to line-up with the protein kinase-like domain of RNase L. Since this domain has been shown to be involved in RNase L homodimerization (30), the cysteine-rich ferredoxin-like structure could introduce a motif in the heterodimeric complex acting as a mock target for RNase L monomers looking for dimerization partners.

Ankyrins constitute a family of proteins containing a consensus repeat sequence which links integral membrane components (by N-terminal interaction) with cytoskeletal elements (by C-terminal interaction) (31). These interactions play fundamental roles in diverse biological activities as they allow to control membrane topology, elasticity and protein composition (32). RLI is an ATP-dependent protein pertaining to the ABC superfamily of transporters, many of which are integral membrane components. Like most members of the ABC superfamily, the amino acid sequence of RLI contains two P-loop consensus motifs, as well as twice the ABC consensus signature pattern (13). Further to these observations, we made a sequence similarity search which delivered significant homologies with several members of the superfamily, as summarized in Figure 3. Many of the identified sequence homologies relate to human multidrug resistance transporters (MDR) and associated proteins (MRP) (33,34). These multidrug transporters bind chemically dissimilar, potentially cytotoxic compounds and remove them from the cell (35). In the absence of cytotoxic agression from external origin, these membrane channels, like ABCE1 (organic anion-binding protein) with which RLI shares 95% identity, mediate the transport of endogenous chemicals such as choline and monoamine neurotransmitters (36). Besides these, RLI sequence shares also homologies with CFTR, SUR1, ABC3, ABC7, ABC8, TAP1 and Rim. CFTR is a chloride channel that regulates anion movement across a transmembrane pore, of which the mutated gene leads to cystic fibrosis (37). CFTR regulates the exocrine function of many epithelial tissues including the pancreas, intestinal glands, biliary tree, bronchial and sweat glands (13). SUR1 takes part of the ATP-sensitive potassium channels (K_{ATP}) of which it regulates the opening function in presence of Mg^{++} (38). SUR1 switches K_{ATP} on or off, depending on the concommitant binding of ATP and ADP (39). Any increase in the ATP/ADP ratio closes the channel which leads to the opening of the voltage-dependent calcium channel. In the β-cell of the pancreas, this mechanism plays a key role in the regulation of glucose-induced insulin secretion. The human ABC3 (homologous to ced-7 of *C. elegans*), plays a key role in the engulfment of cell corpses during apoptosis. It has been proposed that ABC3 functions in both dying and macrophages (engulfing cells) by translocating molecules that mediate homotypic adhesion between the respective cell surfaces (13,26). The ABC7 protein is involved in the transport of heme from the mitochondria to the cytosol (40) and ABC8 is the mammalian homolog of Drosophila white protein (27), involved in eye pigmentation. ABC8 has further been identified as a regulator of macrophage cholesterol and phospholipid transport (41), has been implied in the cellular uptake of tryptophan, a precursor of the neurotransmitter serotonin, and is linked to neurological disorders in humans (42). TAP1 plays a central role in antigen processing and presentation by MHC class I molecules (43). Finally, the absence of retinal specific ABC transporter (ABCR, Rim) in retinal pigment epithelium results in all-trans-retinaldehyde accumulation leading to delayed dark adaptation with secondary photoreceptor degeneration (44). We further show here (see Figure 6) that all these ABC proteins homologous to RLI share with the protein a tetra- or pentapeptide signature which allows ion exchanger proteins (14,15) to interact in the cell cytoplasm with ankyrins.

CFIDS is characterized by debilitating fatigue, muscle and joint pain, as well as several other associated symptoms that are difficult to relate to one another at a physiological level (11). From a biological point of view, the PBMC of patients suffering from the disease contain a small 37-kDa 2-5A-binding protein, which is likely to share the catalytic activity of RNase L (6,7). Experimental evidence from our laboratory indicates that the specific cleavage of the recombinant enzyme by calpain produces some of the same 2-5A-binding proteins observed in CFIDS patients. Calpains are cytosolic cysteine proteases that have been postulated to be involved in cytoskeleton and cell membrane organization and are believed to play key roles in the pathology of disorders such as stroke, Alzheimer's disease, muscular dystrophy, cataract and arthritis (45). Cleavage of r-hRNase L by both calpain and PBMC extracts containing the 37-kDa 2-5A-binding protein results in the release of fragments containing parts of the ankyrin domain (see Figure 2). RLI pertains to the superfamily of ABC transporters and is capable to interact with the ankyrin domain of RNase L (see Figures 4 and 5) through a tetrapeptide motif analogous to that of other ion-exchangers and the interaction precludes the homodimerization of the enzyme. As we show here, the sequence of RLI is strongly homologous to other ABC proteins (see Figure 3) and the homology includes a the tetra- or pentapeptide consensus cluster by which ion channels interact with ankyrin proteins (see Figure 6). Consequently, our results suggest that the ankyrin fragments released from RNase L upon pathological cleavage are able to interact with ABC transporters homologous to RLI, and by competing with their normal cognate ankyrin protein lead to interferences with their normal function. Table 1 summarizes the ABC transporters possibly involved in this abnormal behavior and link their dysfunction with the CFIDS symptoms considered. These results corroborate on biological grounds the clinical observations that had led to this hypothesis (10,12).

Besides extreme debilitating fatigue, the major symptom of CFIDS is unexplained pain. Whilst CFTR has been studied mainly for the mutations responsible for cystic fibrosis (37), its normal function involves the regulation of Na^+ channels (46), which play a major role in the generation of pain and inflammatory hyperalgesia in peripheral neurons (47). In normal conditions, the MDR proteins play a physiological role similar to that of CFTR (48). Consequently, any dysfunction of these ABC transporters leads to a shift of the pain sensitivity threshold. Any such dysfunction in CFTR-Na^+ channel interaction in epithelial cells leads to drenching night sweats as frequently reported by these patients (11). The same dysfunction in MDR leads to the extreme muscle potassium losses and an improper function of SUR1 leads to the transient abnormalities in glucose metabolism as observed in CFIDS (11). A dysfunction in the antigen presentation process by MHC class I resulting from an abnormal TAP1-ankyrin interaction, as well as any interference in the engulfment of apoptotic cells by macrophages resulting from either a metabolic dysregulation due to ABC8, or an ABC3 dysfunction, explains the altered immune function and reactivity as associated with CFIDS (9,11,49). The central nervous system abnormalities observed in CFIDS (11) further find their origin improper activation of either ABC precursor 7 (mutation in the gene leads to ataxia, 40), ABC8 (implied in cellular uptake of tryptophan, a precursor of serotonin, 42), or the Rim protein involved in visual defects (44). The depression which is usually associated with CFIDS (11) can be explained by a dysregulation of the MDR proteins normally involved in monoamine neurotransmitter transport in the brain (36). Finally, a dysfunction in the multidrug resistance proteins (MRP) of which the normal function consists in the terminal excretion of cytotoxic substances (34), explains the hypersensitivity to toxic chemicals associated with CFIDS.

TABLE 1. Summary of the possible links between dysregulated ABC transporters homologous to RLI and CFIDS symptoms.

ABC Transporter (homology with RLI)	Synonym (subfamily)	Physiological role/defect	CFIDS related symptoms
SUR1 (52%)	Sulfonylurea receptor; ABCC8 (MRP/CFTR)	Switches K_{ATP} on/off. In pancreas, regulation of glucose-induced insulin secretion	Transient hypoglycemia
CFTR (49%)	Cystic fibrosis transmembrane conductance regulator ; ABCC7 (MRP/CFTR)	Regulates exocrine function of many epithelial tissues. Interacts with Na^+ channel. Mutation leads to CF	Drenching night sweats Sarcoidosis
MRP6 (47%)	ABCC6 (MRP/CFTR)	Terminal excretion of cytotoxic substances	Hypersensitivity to toxic chemicals.
MRP3 (46%)	ABCC3; MOAT-D (MRP/CFTR)	Terminal excretion of cytotoxic substances	Hypersensitivity to toxic chemicals.
ABC8 (45%)	White homolog; ABCG1 (White)	Eye pigmentation Regulator of macrophage cholesterol and phospholipid homeostasis Tryptophan uptake	Immunodeficiency/Macrophage dysfunction Depression
MDR3 (42%)	Pgp3; ABCB4 (MDR/TAP)	Transport of monoamine neurotransmitters See CFTR	Dysfunction in transport of monoamine neurotransmitter. Pain sensitivity threshold reduced Muscle K^+ loss
TAP1 (42%)	ABCB2 (MDR/TAP)	Processing and presentation of antigens by MHC class I	Immunodeficiency/Th2 switch
ABC7 (40%)	ABCB7 (MDR/TAP)	Transport of heme from mitochondria to cytosol. Mutation leads to ataxia	Anemia CNS abnormalities
ABC3 (40%)	ABCA3; ABC-C (ABC1)	Recognition of apoptotic cells by macrophages for engulfment	Immunodeficiency/Th2 switch
Rim (38%)	ABCR; ABCA4 (ABC1)	Dysfunction leads to all-trans retinaldehyde accumulation	Visual problems

The numerous evidences for links between these currently unexplained CFIDS symptoms and ABC transporter dysfunctions lead us to consider their abnormal interaction with ankyrin fragments released from the pathological cleavage of RNase L as a serious basis for future experimental investigation.

REFERENCES

1. Baglioni, C., Minks, A., Maroney, P. A. Interferon action may be mediated by activation of a nuclease by pppA2'p5'A2'p5'A. *Nature* 1978; *273*: 684-687.

2. Dong, B., Silverman, R. H. 2-5A-dependent RNase molecules dimerize during activation by 2-5A. *J Biol Chem* 1995; *270*: 4133-4137.

3. Aubry, F., Mattéi, M-G., Barque, J. P. et al. Chromosomal localization and expression pattern of the RNase L inhibitor gene. *FEBS Lett* 1996; *381*: 135-139.

4. Bisbal, C., Martinand, C., Silhol, M., et al. Cloning and characterization of a RNase L inhibitor. *J Biol Chem* 1995; *270*: 13308-13317.

5. Dong, B., Silverman, R. H. A bipartite model of 2-5A-dependent RNase L. *J Biol Chem* 1997; *272*: 22236-22242.

6. Suhadolnik, R. J., Peterson, D. L., O'Brien, K. et al. Biochemical evidence for a novel low molecular weight 2-5A-dependent RNase L in chronic fatigue syndrome. *J Interferon Cytokine Res* 1997; *17*: 377-385.

7. Suhadolnik, R. J., Peterson, D. L., Cheney, P. R. et al. Biochemical dysregulation of the 2-5A synthetase/RNase L antiviral defense pathway in chronic fatigue syndrome. *J Chronic Fatigue Syndrome* 1999; *5*: 224-241.

8. De Meirleir, K., Bisbal, C., Campine, I. et al. A 37kDa 2-5A binding protein as a potential biochemical marker for chronic fatigue syndrome. *Am J Med* 2000; *108*: 99-105.

9. Konstantinov, K., von Milkecz, A., Buchwald, D. et al. Autoantibodies to nuclear envelope antigens in chronic fatigue syndrome. *J Clin Invest* 1996; *98*: 1888-1896.

10. Watson, W. S., McCreath, G. T., Chaudhuri, A. et al. Possible cell membrane transport defect in chronic fatigue syndrome? *J Chronic Fatigue Syndrome* 1997; *3*: 1-13.

11. Komaroff A. L., Buchwald, D. S. Chronic fatigue syndrome: an update. *Ann Rev Med* 1998; *49*: 1-13.

12. Chaudhuri, A., Watson, W. S., Pearn, J. et al. The symptoms of chronic fatigue syndrome are related to abnormal ion channel function. *Med Hypotheses* 2000; *54*: 59-63.

13. Klein, I., Sarkadi, B., Varadi, A. An inventory of the human ABC proteins. *Biochim Biophys Acta* 1999; *1461*: 237-262.

14. Jordan, C., Püschel, B., Koob, R. et al. Identification of a binding motif for ankyrin on the α-subunit of Na$^+$, K$^+$-ATPase. *J Biol Chem* 1995; *270*: 29971-29975.

15. Ding, Y., Kobayashi, S., Kopito, R. Mapping of ankyrin binding determinants on the erythroid anion exchanger, AE1. *J Biol Chem* 1996; *271*: 22494-22498.

16. Pearson, W. R. Flexible sequence similarity searching with the FASTA3 program package. *Methods Mol Biol* 2000; *132*: 185-219.

17. Altschul, S. F., Madden, T. L., Schäffer, A. A. et al. Gapped BLAST and PSI-BLAST: a new generation of protein database search programs. *Nucleic Acids Res* 1997; *25*: 3389-3402.

18. Guex, N., Peitsch, M. C. SWISS-MODEL and the Swiss-Pdb viewer: an environment for comparative protein modeling. *Electrophoresis* 1997; *18*: 2714-2723.

19. Guex, N., Diemand, A., Peitsch, M. C. Protein modelling for all. *Trends Biochem Sci* 1999; *24*: 364-367.

20. Abagyan, R. A., Trotov, M. M., Kuznetsov, D. N. ICM–a new method for protein modeling and design. Applications to docking and structure prediction from the distorted native conformation. *J Comp Chem* 1994; *15*: 488-506.

21. Thompson, J. D., Higgins, D. G., Gibson, T. J. CLUSTAL W: improving the sensitivity of progressive multiple sequence alignment through sequence weighting, position-specific gap penalties and weight matrix choice. *Nucleic Acids Res* 1994; *22*: 4673-4680.

22. Zhou, A., Hassel, B. A., Silverman, R. H. Expression cloning of 2-5A-dependent RNAase: a uniquely regulated mediator of interferon action. *Cell* 1993; *72*: 753-765.

23. Lux, S. E., John, K. M., Bennett, V. Analysis of cDNA for human erythrocyte ankyrin indicates a repeated structure with homology to tissue-differentiation and cell-cycle control proteins. *Nature* 1990; *344*: 36-42.

24. Tsai, M. J., O'Malley, B. W. Molecular mechanisms of action of steroid/thyroid receptor superfamily members. *Annu Rev Biochem* 1994; *402*: 451-486.

25. Hyde, S. C., Emsley, P., Hartshorn, M. J. et al. Structural model of ATP-binding proteins associated with cystic fibrosis, multidrug resistance and bacterial transport. *Nature* 1990; *346*: 362-365.

26. Broccardo, C., Luciani, M-F., Chimini, G. The ABCA subclass of mammalian transporters. *Biochim Biophys Acta* 1999; *1461*: 395-404.

27. Savary, S., Denizot, F., Luciani, M. et al. Molecular cloning of a mammalian ABC transporter homologous to Drosophila white gene. *Mamm. Genome* 1996; *7*: 673-676.

28. Rozet, J. M., Gerber, S., Souied, E. et al. The ABCR gene: a major disease gene in macular and peripheral retinal degenerations with onset from early childhood to the elderly. *Mol Genet Metab* 1999; *68*: 310-315.

29. Zhang, Z., Devarajan, P., Dorfman, A. L. et al. Structure of the ankyrin-binding domain of α-Na, K-ATPase. *J Biol Chem* 1998; *273*: 18681-18684.

30. Dong, B., Silverman, R. H. Alternative function of a protein kinase homology domain in 2′,5′-oligoadenylate dependent RNase L. *Nucleic Acids Res* 1999; *27*: 439-445.

31. Bennett, V., Otto, E., Kunimoto, M. et al. Diversity of ankyrins in the brain. *Biochem Soc Trans* 1991; *19*: 1034-1039.

32. Michaely, P., Kamal, A., Anderson, R. G. W. et al. A requirement for ankyrin binding to clathrin during coated pit budding. *J Biol Chem* 1999; *274*: 35908-35913.

33. Klugbauer, N., Hofmann, F. Primary structure of a novel ABC transporter with a chromosomal localization on the band encoding the multidrug resistance-associated protein. *FEBS Lett* 1996; *391*: 61-65.

34. Konig, J., Nies, A. T., Cui, Y. et al. Conjugate export pumps of the multidrug resistance protein (MRP) family: localization, substrate specificity, and MRP2-mediated drug resistance. *Biochim Biophys Acta* 1999; *1461*: 377-394.

35. Zheleznova, E. E., Markham, P., Edgar, R. et al. A structure-based mechanism for drug binding by multidrug transporters. *Trends Biochem Sci* 2000; *25*, 39-43.

36. Koepsell, H. Organic cation transporters in intestine, kidney, liver and brain. *Annu Rev Physiol* 1998; *60*: 243-266.

37. Seibert, F. S., Jia, Y., Mathews, C. J. et al. Disease-associated mutations in cytoplasmic loops 1 and 2 of cystic fibrosis transmembrane conductance regulator impede processing or opening of the channel. *Biochem* 1997; *36,* 11966-11974.

38. Schwanstecher, M., Sieverding, C., Dorschner, H. et al. Potassium channel openers require ATP to bind to and act through sulfonylurea receptors. *EMBO J* 1998; *17*: 5529-5535.

39. Ueda, K., Matsuo, M., Tanabe, K. et al. Comparative aspects of the function and mechanism of SUR1 and MDR1 proteins. *Biochim Biophys Acta* 1999; *1461*: 305-313.

40. Allikmets, R., Raskind, W. H., Hutchinson, A. et al. Mutation of a putative mitochondrial iron transporter gene (ABC7) in X-linked sideroblastic anemia and ataxia (XLSA/A). *Hum Mol Genet* 1999; *8*: 743-749.

41. Klucken, J., Buchler, C., Orso, E. et al. ABCG1 (ABC8), the human homolog of the Drosophila white gene, is a regulator of macrophage cholesterol and phospholipid transport. *Proc Nat Acad Sci USA* 2000; *97*: 817-822.

42. Croop, J. M., Tiller, G. E., Fletcher, J. A. et al. Isolation and characterization of a mammalian homolog of the Drosophila white gene. *Gene* 1997; *185,* 77-85.

43. Creswell, P., Bangia, N., Dick, T. et al. The nature of the MHC class I peptide loading complex. *Immunol Rev* 1999; *172*: 21-28.

44. Weng, J., Mata, N. L., Azarian, S. M. et al. Insights into the function of Rim protein in photoreceptors and etiology of Stargardt's disease from the phenotype in abcr knockout mice. *Cell* 1999; *98*: 13-23.

45. Leung, D., Abbenante, G., Fairlie, D. P. Protease inhibitors: current status and future prospects. *J Med Chem* 2000; *43*: 305-341.

46. Kunzelmann, K., Schreiber, R. CFTR, a regulator of channels. *J Membr Biol* 1999; *168*: 1-8.

47. Dubner, R., Gold, M. The neurobiology of pain. *Proc Natl Acad Sci USA* 1999; *96*: 7627-7630.

48. Valverde, M. A., Diaz, M., Sepulveda, F. V. et al. Volume-regulated chloride channels associated with the human multidrug-resistance P-glycoprotein. *Nature* 1992; *355*: 830-833.

49. Vedhara, K., Llewelyn, M. B., Fox, J. D. et al. Consequences of live poliovirus vaccine administration in chronic fatigue syndrome. *J Neuroimmunol* 1997; *75*: 183-195.

Assessment of Functional Impairment by Cardiopulmonary Exercise Testing in Patients with Chronic Fatigue Syndrome

J. Mark VanNess, PhD
Christopher R. Snell, PhD
Dean M. Fredrickson, BS
David R. Strayer, MD
Staci R. Stevens, MA

SUMMARY. Functional impairment in a population of patients with chronic fatigue syndrome (CFS) was determined by exercise testing. The criteria established by Weber and Janicki (1) were employed because impairment levels are based on maximal oxygen consumption. Oxygen consumption was obtained by cardiopulmonary exercise testing and was used to classify subjects according to the severity of impairment. All the

J. Mark VanNess and Christopher R. Snell are affiliated with the Department of Sport Sciences, University of the Pacific, 3601 Pacific Avenue, Stockton, CA 95211-0197.

David R. Strayer is affiliated with Hemispherx Biopharma, 1617 JFK Boulevard, Philladelphia, PA 19103.

Staci R. Stevens and Dean M. Fredrickson are affiliated with the Workwell Foundation, P.O. Box 114, Ripon, CA 95366.

Address correspondence to: J. Mark VanNess, PhD, Department of Sport Sciences, University of the Pacific, 3601 Pacific Avenue, Stockton, CA 95211-0197.

The authors thank the following for their valuable contributions to this research project: Joseph R. Bellesorte, DO; Daniel L. Peterson, MD; Paul J. Cimoch, MD; Richard N. Podell, MD; Joseph F. John, MD; James L. Sepoil, MD; Robert H. Keller, MD, FACP; Bruce E. Stein, MD; Alex Mercandetti, MD; Leslie H. Taylor, MD; Mary M. Eberhart; and William A. Carter, MD.

[Haworth co-indexing entry note]: "Assessment of Functional Impairment by Cardiopulmonary Exercise Testing in Patients with Chronic Fatigue Syndrome." VanNess, J. Mark et al. Co-published simultaneously in *Journal of Chronic Fatigue Syndrome* (The Haworth Medical Press, an imprint of The Haworth Press, Inc.) Vol. 8, No. 3/4, 2001, pp. 103-109; and: *Innovations in Chronic Fatigue Syndrome Research and Clinical Practice* (ed: Roberto Patarca-Montero) The Haworth Medical Press, an imprint of The Haworth Press, Inc., 2001, pp. 103-109. Single or multiple copies of this article are available for a fee from The Haworth Document Delivery Service [1-800-342-9678, 9:00 a.m. - 5:00 p.m. (EST). E-mail address: getinfo@haworthpressinc.com].

"

subjects in this study met the CDC case definition (2) for CFS. All patients underwent at least two maximal graded exercise tests in which expired air was collected for assessment of VO_2max. Data are included for eighty-seven CFS patients, the highest VO_2 was used for determining impairment. Although all patients met the CDC case definition for CFS, only 35 (40%) would be classified as having greater than "Mild" functional impairment. The highest VO_2 of any of the patients in this study was 29.5 ml/kg/min, very close to what normative data predicts to be the average maximal value for the entire group. Without a sedentary control group it is unclear if the low VO_2 in this population is due to the pathology of CFS or results from the inactivity that accompanies the disease. However, use of maximal VO_2 during exercise can clearly discriminate between levels of functional impairment and may be efficacious for diagnosis of CFS. Additionally, in cases where cardiopulmonary analysis is unavailable, exercise duration on a standardized test may also be employed. *[Article copies available for a fee from The Haworth Document Delivery Service: 1-800-342-9678. E-mail address: <getinfo@haworthpressinc.com> Website: <http://www.HaworthPress.com> © 2001 by The Haworth Press, Inc. All rights reserved.]*

KEYWORDS. Chronic fatigue syndrome, cardiopulmonary exercise testing, disability assessment, functional impairment, oxygen consumption

INTRODUCTION

Chronic fatigue syndrome (CFS) is an illness characterized by profound debilitating fatigue which dramatically reduces a person's ability to carry out even normal daily activities. Diagnosis of CFS relies in part on the subjective comparison of present levels of fatigue and functional capacity with levels prior to disease onset. Quantifying fatigue in CFS is difficult because it is experienced differently by each patient. The subjective nature of fatigue and its effects also presents problems when assessing the efficacy of therapeutic strategies and pharmacological interventions designed to relieve the symptoms that accompany CFS.

Cardiopulmonary analysis during a graded exercise test can provide an objective assessment of the effects of CFS on functional capacity by the measurement of oxygen consumption. Oxygen consumption, or the volume of oxygen a person can use in the process of energy production (VO_2), is the result of the integrated actions of the cardiovascular, metabolic, and respiratory systems. VO_2 can provide an objective assessment of the ability to perform physical work and to determine level of impairment. By providing an objective measure of exercise capacity, cardiopulmonary exercise testing is of considerable value in disability assessment. In addition to disability evaluation, exercise testing can be used for differential diagnosis and for assessment of improved functional capacity following drug therapy and rehabilitation. Exercise testing is often used to determine the level of impairment associated with a number of chronic diseases such as cardiac and vascular failure, pulmonary disorders, and mitochondrial enzyme defects. We propose that exercise testing techniques can be similarly applied to disability assessment for CFS.

The purpose of this study was therefore to determine peak oxygen consumption in a patient population with confirmed diagnosis of CFS, and compare these values to previously established criteria for functional impairment.

METHODS

Subjects

The subjects for this study were eighty-seven patients with CFS (62 females and 25 males age: 45 ± 1 years). Only individuals with a confirmed and rigorous diagnosis of CFS according to the criteria established by Holmes et al. (2) and Fukuda et al. (3) participated in the study. Individuals with concurrent medical disorders, or who had been treated with drugs that modulate the immune, cardiovascular, or respiratory systems within six weeks of testing were excluded from the study. Additionally, the investigators excluded from the study patients with prominent psychological or medical disorders that may have interfered with their ability to perform the graded exercise test. All subjects signed an informed consent document prior to beginning testing. Subjects were instructed to avoid food, alcohol, and caffeine for at least three hours prior to testing, they were also asked to avoid significant exertion or exercise for 24 hours prior to testing. Data were collected by exercise physiologists at nine testing sites across the United States.

Cardiopulmonary Graded Exercise Test

The entire procedure for exercise testing was explained in detail to each patient prior to testing. Subjects were fitted with ECG electrodes (Lynn Medical; 650-030) for monitoring of heart rhythm, a mask and headgear (Hans Rudolph) for collection of expired air, and a pulse oximeter (Nelcor N-200) for monitoring arterial oxygen saturation. All subjects were allowed to walk briefly (less than one minute) on the treadmill (Trackmaster; TM225T) to allow them to feel comfortable. The following exercise protocol was followed:

Time	Speed	Grade
0-2 min	2 mph	0%
2-4 min	2 mph	3%
4-6 min	2 mph	6%
6-8 min	2 mph	9%
8-10 min	2 mph	12%
10-12 min	2 mph	15%
12-14 min	2 mph	18%
14-16 min	2 mph	21%
16-18 min	3 mph	21%
18-20 min	4 mph	21%
20-22 min	5 mph	21%

Oxygen consumption was measured breath by breath, rating of perceived exertion (RPE; Borg Scale) was collected every minute, and blood pressure was taken manually every two minutes.

Exercise continued either to volitional fatigue, until the subject could no longer maintain position on the treadmill, or the test technician stopped the test to comply with ACSM guidelines. All patients performed at least two exercise tests, two weeks apart. A third test was required if duration for the first two tests differed by more than 10%. The highest value for peak oxygen consumption obtained from the tests is reported.

Data Analysis

Values recorded for peak oxygen consumption where compared with the severity of impairment index developed by Weber and Janicki (1) which utilizes maximal oxygen consumption (VO_2max) to quantify level of disability.

RESULTS

Data are included for eighty-seven CFS patients (62 females and 25 males, 45 ± 1 years), the highest VO_2 values were used to determine impairment level. The number of patients at each level along with group means $\pm$ standard error for peak VO_2 and exercise duration are presented below in Table 1.

Although all patients met the CDC case definition for CFS, only 35 (40%) would be classified as having greater than "Mild" functional impairment. The highest VO_2 of any of the patients in this study was 29.5 ml/kg/min, very close to what normative data predicts should be the average maximal value for the entire group.

CONCLUSIONS

The ability of these CFS patients to undertake two or three graded exercise tests supports the viability of exercise testing for disability assessment in this population. Other research examining exercise testing and CFS indicates a high level of consistency between repeated exercise tests which suggests that even a single graded exercise test may be a reliable measure of performance for CFS patients (4).

A number of studies looking at exercise capacity in CFS patients have failed to report reduced performance (e.g., 5,6). However, the results of this study would seem to concur with yet other research that has demonstrated reduced oxygen consumption and reduced exercise capacity in CFS patients (e.g., 7,8). While diminished exercise capacity was readily apparent in these CFS patients, without a sedentary control

TABLE 1

Severity of Impairment	Peak VO_2 ml/kg/min	# of Patients	Group VO_2 ml/kg/min	Exercise Duration (min)
None	>25	7	28.5 ± 1.2	$15:30 \pm 0:46$
Mild	20-25	36	22.4 ± 0.2	$13:05 \pm 0:26$
Moderate	15-20	25	18.1 ± 0.3	$9:59 \pm 0:33$
Severe	<15	10	12.5 ± 0.6	$5:15 \pm 0:50$

group it is unclear if the low VO_2 in this population is due to the pathology of CFS or results from the inactivity that accompanies the disease.

Despite this uncertainty over the etiology of fatigue in CFS graded exercise testing is still useful as a measure of impairment. It should also provide an objective assessment of any improvement in function following treatment (which could include reconditioning) or, conversely, degeneration as a consequence of disease progression.

When employing exercise testing to assess impairment in CFS patients it is important to note that persons with CFS have been shown to be incapable of performing a maximal test as defined for normal populations (8,9). Accepted criteria to denote a maximal test include respiratory exchange ratio greater than 1.0, attainment of age predicted maximal heart rate, and plateau or decline of VO_2 at the final workloads. Observation of one to all of these criteria may be required as confirmation of a maximal test. Certain of these criteria are particularly problematic for CFS because of symptoms associated with the disease. This is especially the case for attainment of age predicted maximal heart rate since cardiac autonomic balance is impaired in this population (10). Using the highest value of all tests in the analysis along with at least one other of the accepted criteria maximizes the likelihood that all values recorded reflect maximal performance.

A further point of interest concerns the variability between individuals with respect to level of impairment. This reinforces the complex nature of CFS and may even indicate multiple origins for the pathology of CFS as currently defined. Further research to explore energy metabolism during exercise may help reveal or confirm the cellular basis of fatigue in CFS.

REFERENCES

1. Weber KT, Janicki JS (1986). Cardiopulmonary exercise testing: physiologic principles and clinical applications. Philadelphia: W. B. Saunders Company.

2. Holmes GP, Kaplan JE, Schonberger LB. Definition of the chronic fatigue syndrome. *Annals of Internal Medicine* 1988; 109: 512-522.

3. Fukuda K, Straus SE, Hickie I, Sharpe MC, Dobbins JG, Komaroff A. Chronic fatigue syndrome: a comprehensive approach to its definition and study. *Annals of Internal Medicine* 1994; 121: 953-959.

4. Snell CR, VanNess JM, Fredrickson DM, Strayer DR, Treutler K, LaRosa E, Stevens SR, and AMP-516 Investigators. Variability of repeated exercise testing in patients with chronic fatigue syndrome. *Federation of the American Society for Experimental Biology Journal* 2000; 14 (4): LB42.

5. Edwards R, Gibson H, Clague J, Helliwell T. Muscle histopathology and physiology in chronic fatigue syndrome. *Ciba Foundation Symposium* 1993; 173: 102-117.

6. Sisto SA, LaManca J, Cordero DL, Bergen MT, Ellis SP, Drastal S, Boda DL, Tapp WN, Natelson BH. Metabolic and cardiovascular effects of a progressive exercise test in patients with chronic fatigue syndrome. *American Journal of Medicine* 1996; 100: 634-640.

7. Riley MS, O'Brien CJ, McCloskey DR, Bell NP, Nicholls DP. Aerobic work capacity in patients with chronic fatigue syndrome. *British Medical Journal* 1990; 301: 953-956.

8. Make B, Jones JF. Impairment of patients with chronic fatigue syndrome. *Journal of Chronic Fatigue Syndrome* 1997; 3 (4): 43-55.

9. VanNess JM, Snell CR, Fredrickson DM, Strayer DR, LaRosa E, Treutler K, Stevens SR. Exercise testing in patients with chronic fatigue syndrome (CFS)–Diagnostic tool? *Federation of the American Society for Experimental Biology Journal* 2000; 14 (4): LB41.

10. Farrar D, Locke S, Kantrowitz F. Chronic fatigue syndrome 1: Etiology and pathogenesis. *Behavioral Medicine* 1995; 21: 1-16.

Hypercoaguable State Associated with Active Human Herpesvirus-6 (HHV-6) Viremia in Patients with Chronic Fatigue Syndrome

Joseph H. Brewer, MD
David Berg, MS

SUMMARY. Objectives: A subset of patients with Chronic Fatigue Syndrome (CFS) have been found to be hypercoaguable in small previous studies. We wanted to analyze the incidence of a hypercoaguable state and assess hereditary hypercoaguable risk factors in a group of patients with known CFS and HHV-6 viremia.

Methods: Thirty patients diagnosed with CFS that had at least one prior positive blood culture for active HHV-6 by rapid culture method were studied. A hypercoaguable panel was obtained to assess activation of coagulation. Two or more positive tests were determined to represent activation of coagulation. Hereditary thrombosis risk panels were also performed which included eight different genetic tests to assess hereditary abnormalities.

Results: Twenty-four of thirty (80%) patients had a hypercoaguable state, thus activation of coagulation. Twenty-five of thirty (83%) of patients had a hereditary abnormality.

Joseph H. Brewer is affiliated with Plaza Internal Medicine-Infectious Disease and St. Luke's Hospital (Infectious Diseases) in Kansas City, MO.

David Berg is Director, Hemex Labortories, Phoenix, AZ.

Address correspondence to: Joseph H. Brewer, MD, 4620 J. C. Nichols Parkway, Suite 415, Kansas City, MO 64112.

[Haworth co-indexing entry note]: "Hypercoaguable State Associated with Active Human Herpesvirus-6 (HHV-6) Viremia in Patients with Chronic Fatigue Syndrome." Brewer, Joseph H., and David Berg. Co-published simultaneously in *Journal of Chronic Fatigue Syndrome* (The Haworth Medical Press, an imprint of The Haworth Press, Inc.) Vol. 8, No. 3/4, 2001, pp. 111-116; and: *Innovations in Chronic Fatigue Syndrome Research and Clinical Practice* (ed: Roberto Patarca-Montero) The Haworth Medical Press, an imprint of The Haworth Press, Inc., 2001, pp. 111-116. Single or multiple copies of this article are available for a fee from The Haworth Document Delivery Service [1-800-342-9678, 9:00 a.m. - 5:00 p.m. (EST). E-mail address: getinfo@haworthpressinc.com].

Conclusions: CFS patients with active HHV-6 infection (viremia) have activation of coagulation and are hypercoaguable. Hereditary thrombosis risk factors are very prevalent in these patients. These hereditary abnormalities increase the hypercoaguable tendencies. The hypercoaguable state associated with active HHV-6 infection may be a significant contributing factor to the symptoms seen in CFS patients. *[Article copies available for a fee from The Haworth Document Delivery Service: 1-800-342-9678. E-mail address: <getinfo@haworthpressinc.com> Website: <http://www. HaworthPress.com> © 2001 by The Haworth Press, Inc. All rights reserved.]*

KEYWORDS. Chronic fatigue syndrome (CFS), human herpesvirus-6 (HHV-6), hypercoaguable syndrome, hereditary thrombosis risk

INTRODUCTION

An association with active human herpesvirus-6 (HHV-6) infection and chronic fatigue syndrome (CFS) has been reported in several studies (1-3). Utilizing a rapid blood culture technique, active infection with HHV-6 (viremia) was found in 30-70% of CFS patients compared to healthy controls in which no positive cultures were found (3). In a study of 20 CFS patients, a significant proportion was to shown to be hypercoaguable as compared to healthy controls (4). A hypercoaguable syndrome in CFS patients may explain many of the symptoms due to diminished oxygen delivery to tissues as well as diminished venous outflow from tissues.

In this study, we selectively looked at a group of patients with CFS who had HHV-6 viremia as demonstrated by a positive blood culture. We assessed the presence and frequency of a hypercoaguable syndrome in these patients by analyzing several different coagulation parameters. Additionally, we analyzed the incidence of hereditary hypercoaguable/thrombosis risk factors by testing for eight different genetic traits.

METHODS

Thirty patients (25 female, 5 male) from one medical practice were studied. All patients satisfied the Centers for Disease Control case definition for CFS (5). All 30 patients previously had at least one positive blood culture for active HHV-6 utilizing the rapid blood culture previously described (6). A hypercoaguable panel (previously described as the ISAC panel) was performed on blood specimens from each of the 30 patients (4). The hypercoaguable (ISAC) panel to assess activation of coagulation included the following tests: fibrinogen level (FB), pro-thrombin fragments 1 + 2 (PF 1 + 2), thrombin/antithrombin complexes (T/AT), soluble fibrin monomer (SFM), and platelet activation (PL Act) by flow cytometry. Two or more positive tests from this panel were determined to represent evidence of a hypercoaguable state and activation of coagulation. Hereditary thrombosis risk panels were also performed on all 30 patients. These tests included: antithrombin activity (AT), protein C activity (PC), protein S activity (PS), activated protein C resistance assay (APCR), factor II activity (F II), homocysteine level (HC), lipoprotein (a) level (Lp(a)) and plasminogen activator inhibi-tor-1 level (PAI-1). All coagulation testing was done at Hemex Labora-tories. All blood specimens were drawn first AM, fasting. None of the patients were on anticoagulant therapy.

RESULTS

The results of hypercaguable testing and hereditary testing are sum-marized in Tables 1 and 2.

DISCUSSION

CFS has been associated with active HHV-6 infection (1-3). It may well be that active infection with this virus plays a key role in the pathogenesis of CFS and symptom production. An abnormal ISAC panel, indicating a hypercoaguable state and activation of coagulation, was seen in 24 of 30 (80%) of CFS/HHV-6 patients. This activation likely leads to fibrin formation and deposition in blood vessels. The mechanism for activation of the coagulation system in these patients is unclear but may involve active infection and the inflammatory re-sponse. HHV-6 has been clearly shown to infect endothelial cells (7-9). The effect of active HHV-6 infection on endothelial cell function is un-known. HHV-6, when activated, may give rise to enhanced proco-agulant activity and thus a hypercoaguable syndrome. Several studies have shown a definite procoagulant effect of cytomegalovirus (CMV) on endothelial cells (10-12). Among the herpesvirus family, HHV-6 and CMV are closely related (13). Similar to what has been described previously with CMV, we suggest that HHV-6 infection of endothelial

TABLE 1. Hypercoaguable Testing (ISAC Panel)

	No.	FB	PF1+2	T/AT	SFM	PL Act	>2 abnorm.
M	5	1	3	1	3	3	3
F	25	11	12	3	14	9	21
Total	30	12	15	4	17	13	24
%		40	50	13	57	43	80

Abbreviations: M–male, F–female, FB–fibrinogen level, PT1 + 2–prothrombin fragments 1 + 2, T/AT–thrombin/antithrombin complexes, SFM–soluble fibrin monomer, PL act–platelet activation

TABLE 2. Hereditary Hypercoaguable Traits

	No.	AT	PC	PS	F II	Lp(a)	PAI-1	HC	1 abnorm.	> 1 abnorm.
M	5	0	0	0	1	2	2	2	4	2
F	25	0	0	3	8	9	9	8	21	14
Total (n)	30	0	0	3	9	11	11	10	25	16
%		0	0	10	30	37	37	33	83	53

Abbreviations: M–male, F–female, AT antithrombin level, PC–protein C level, PS–protein S level, F II–factor II level, Lp(a)–lipoprotein (a) level, PAI-1–plasminogen activator inhibitor-1 level, HC homocysteine level

cells may result in a procoagulant effect on the endothelial cell. Active HHV-6 infection of endothelial cells may induce dysfunction of these cells and disrupt the balance between the procoagulant tendency and natural anticoagulant activity. This leads to fibrin deposition, increased blood viscosity and diminished flow.

Previous data collected by one of us (Berg) has shown a high incidence of hereditary abnormalities in the vast majority (> 80%) of 20 patients with CFS studied (unpublished observations). In the present study, when we tested for 8 different hereditary hypercoaguable traits, we found strikingly similar results to those previous findings. In our study, 25 of 30 patients (83%) with CFS and HHV-6 viremia had at least one hereditary coagulation abnormality. Two or more hereditary abnormalities were found in 16 of 30 (53%) of these patients. It is estimated that thirty percent of blood proteins are involved with regulation of coagulation. As a result of mutational defects in these proteins, approximately 5% of the population have bleeding defects and 20% or more have clotting defects. The finding that over 80% of patients with CFS and active HHV-6 infection have a hereditary hypercoaguable trait is intriguing. This data suggests that patients with hereditary hyper-coaguable traits have increased risk for developing CFS symptoms in the setting of HHV-6 activation (reactivation). We propose that active HHV-6 infection of endothelial cells gives rise to transient endothelial cell dysfunction and increased procoagulant activity, thus activation of coagulation. Such active infection may or may not induce circulatory abnormalities based on the severity and duration of active viral infection and resultant endothelial cell dysfunction. In the setting of a hypercoaguable hereditary disorder, the procoagulant state and activation of coagulation may be substantially amplified leading to more pronounced circulatory compromise. With regard to the hereditary thrombophilia traits, we only found decreased PS and increased F II levels in this group of patients. Whether the increased F II levels are related to a prothrombin gene mutation or not, is unclear, since we did not specifically test for that mutation. Interestingly, we found a high percentage of patients had hereditary hypofibrinolysis abnormalities (Lp(a), PAI-1, HC). This suggests that these patients have a hypercoaguable syndrome with active fibrin deposition but they are unable to appropriately initiate fibrinolysis and "keep pace" with the fibrin deposition.

This model of a hypercoaguable syndrome in CFS patients with active HHV-6 infection should be further investigated. It raises several important questions regarding treatment of the active virus infection and anticoagulation as management strategies for CFS patients.

CONCLUSION

Active infection with HHV-6 has been demonstrated among patients with CFS. In small studies, a significant proportion of patients have also been shown to have a hypercoaguable syndrome. In this study of patients with CFS and active HHV-6 infection, we found that 80% are hypercoaguable (positive ISAC panel) and 83% have a hereditary hypercoaguable abnormality (at least one abnormal trait). Since HHV-6 is known to infect endothelial cells, there may be a resultant endothelial cell dysfunction triggering the coagulation system, similar to the procoagulant effect that has been described with CMV. The hereditary hypercoaguable abnormalities may indeed further tip the balance toward an amplification of the hypercoaguable syndrome. Recognition of the activation of coagulation and the hereditary hypercoaguable abnormalities in these patients with active HHV-6 viremia may be important in our understanding of this syndrome and the management of these patients.

REFERENCES

1. Buchwald D, Cheney PR, Peterson DL et al. A chronic illness characterized by fatigue, neurologic and immunologic disorders, and active human herpesvirus type 6 infection. Ann Intern Med 1992; 116: 103-113.

2. Zorenzenon M, Rukh G, Botta GA et al. Active HHV-6 infection in chronic fatigue syndrome patients from Italy: New data. J Chron Fatigue Syndr 1996; 2 (4): 3-12.

3. Knox KK, Brewer JH, and Carrigan DR. Persistent active human herpesvirus six (HHV-6) infections in patients with chronic fatigue syndrome. J Chron Fatigue Syndr 1999; 5(3/4): 245-246.

4. Berg D, Berg LH, Couvarars J. Is CFS associated with an undefined hypercoaguable state brought on by immune activation of coagulation? J Chron Fatigue Syndr 1999; 5(3/4): 113-114.

5. Fikuda K, Strauss SE, Hickie I et al. The chronic fatigue syndrome: A comprehensive approach to its definition and study. Ann Intern Med 1994; 121: 953-959.

6. Knox KK, Brewer JH, Henry JM et al. Human herpesvirus 6 and multiple sclerosis: Systemic active infections in patients with early disease. Clin Infect Dis 2000: 31: 894-903.

7. Wu CA, Shanley JD. Chronic infection of human umbilical vein endothelial cells by human herpesvirus-6. J Gen Virol 1998; 79: 1247-1256.

8. Ueda T, Miyake Y, Imoto K et al. Distribution of human herpesvirus 6 and varicellazoster virus in organs of a fatal case with exanthem subitum and varicella. Acta Paediatr Jpn 1996; 38: 590-595.

9. Rotola A, DiLuca D, Cassai E et al. Human herpesvirus 6 infects and replicates in aortic endothelium. J Clin Microbiol 2000; 38: 3135-3136.

10. Brvggerman CA, Debie WM, Grauls G et al. Cytomegalovirus infection of rat endothelial cells *in vitro*. Arch Virol 1986; 87: 265-272.

11. Van Dam-Mieraras MC, Bruggman CA, Muller AD et al. Induction of endothelial cell procoagulant activity by cytomegalovirus infection. Thromb Res 1987; 47: 69-75.

12. Van Dam-Mieras MC, Muller AD, Van Hinsbergh VW et al. The procoagulant response of cytomegalovirus infected endothelial cells. Thromb Haemost 1992; 68: 364-370.

13. Braun DK, Dominguez G, Pellet PE. Human herpesvirvs 6. Clin Microbiol Rev 1997; 10: 521-567.

Chronic Fatigue Syndrome, Ampligen, and Quality of Life: A Phenomenological Perspective

Christopher R. Snell, PhD
Staci R. Stevens, MA
J. Mark VanNess, PhD

SUMMARY. The purpose of this investigation was to identify significant quality-of-life issues for two women previously diagnosed with chronic fatigue syndrome (CFS), and their families. Both women were participants in a cost-recovery, clinical trial of the antiviral and immunomodulatory drug, Ampligen.

A qualitative, case study approach was adopted to access information not normally available from clinical trials. Specifically, semi-structured, in-depth interviews were conducted with the CFS patients, and their spouses, to discover if these families perceived any changes in their patterns of daily living contingent with participation in the Ampligen trial. Patient diaries were also analyzed for the purpose of triangulation.

Content analysis of the interview transcripts and diary entries revealed a number of significant quality of life improvements for the women and their families, for which they perceived the drug therapy responsible. After an initial acclimation period, and with the exception of

Christopher R. Snell and J. Mark VanNess are affiliated with the Department of Sport Sciences, University of the Pacific, 3601 Pacific Avenue, Stockton, CA 95211-0197.

Staci R. Stevens is affiliated with the Workwell Foundation, P.O. Box 114, Ripon, CA 95366.

Address correspondence to: J. Mark VanNess, PhD, Department of Sport Sciences, University of the Pacific, 3601 Pacific Avenue, Stockton, CA 95211-0197.

[Haworth co-indexing entry note]: "Chronic Fatigue Syndrome, Ampligen, and Quality of Life: A Phenomenological Perspective." Snell, Christopher, R., Staci R. Stevens, and J. Mark VanNess. Co-published simultaneously in *Journal of Chronic Fatigue Syndrome* (The Haworth Medical Press, an imprint of The Haworth Press, Inc.) Vol. 8, No. 3/4, 2001, pp. 117-121; and: *Innovations in Chronic Fatigue Syndrome Research and Clinical Practice* (ed: Roberto Patarca-Montero) The Haworth Medical Press, an imprint of The Haworth Press, Inc., 2001, pp. 117-121. Single or multiple copies of this article are available for a fee from The Haworth Document Delivery Service [1-800-342-9678, 9:00 a.m. - 5:00 p.m. (EST). E-mail address: getinfo@haworthpressinc.com].

the day when the drug was administered, both women reported a reduction in pain, increased energy levels, and improved cognitive functioning. They each cited numerous cases to illustrate their improvement. *[Article copies available for a fee from The Haworth Document Delivery Service: 1-800-342-9678. E-mail address: <getinfo@haworthpressinc.com> Website: <http://www.HaworthPress.com> © 2001 by The Haworth Press, Inc. All rights reserved.]*

KEYWORDS. Chronic fatigue syndrome, quality of life, Ampligen, qualitative research

INTRODUCTION

Because of the dramatic changes in a person's quality of life contingent with the onset of Chronic Fatigue Syndrome (CFS), any potential treatment that can ameliorate the symptoms of the disease and restore some element of normalcy to the daily existence of CFS patients is of great significance to these individuals and all those interested in CFS. The primary purpose of this paper is to describe the response of two long-time CFS sufferers to treatment with the drug Ampligen (poly I:poly $C_{12}U$).

Ampligen is a specific form of mismatched, double-stranded ribonucleic acid (dsRNA) with antiviral and immune modulatory properties that has been effective in providing long-lasting clinical benefit to severely afflicted CFS patients (1). While the etiology and mechanisms of CFS are still the subject of much debate, persistent viral infection and immune system dysfunction are pathologies common to many CFS patients (2). There is evidence to suggest that the viral defense pathways of certain CFS patients are significantly impaired and that viral disruption of energy metabolism may be the cellular basis of fatigue in CFS (3,4). The effectiveness of an immunomodulatory drug such as Ampligen does lend some support to this hypothesis.

The phenomenological perspective adopted here details the experiences of two women participating in a cost-recovery, clinical trial of the drug, both of whom believe that Ampligen therapy has resulted in significantly improved quality of life for them and their families. The self-reported improvements in the quality of life now experienced by these women might even be interpreted as evidence of remission from CFS.

METHODS

Phenomenological methodologies view situations from the perspectives of the participants. Such qualitative research strategies can be particularly useful for exploring diseases where patient symptoms are often subjective and self-reported. Patient interviews commonly provide much of the data for case studies in CFS (5). Increasingly phenomenological methods are being advocated when it is important to consider symptoms like fatigue in the context of patient's daily lives (6,7).

For this study a qualitative, case-study approach was adopted to access information not normally available from clinical trials. Specifically, semi-structured, in-depth interviews were conducted with two female CFS patients, and their spouses, to discover if these families perceived any changes in their patterns of daily living since becoming involved in the Ampligen trial. Patient diaries were also analyzed to provide further insights into the lives of these people.

RESULTS AND DISCUSSION

The first study participant is a 49-year-old women who has suffered with CFS since 1989. As a very active individual prior to contracting the disease, she had found the limitations imposed by CFS particularly difficult to accept. In an earlier interview she reported some progress in managing the disease through the adoption of strategies for conserving energy and a prescribed exercise program comprised of short-duration activities designed to increase strength and flexibility. This had made her feel "empowered" and less "victimized" by the disease, which had helped restore her self-image while reducing the experience of muscle and joint pain (8). At the time of this first interview she had just begun involvement in the Ampligen trial.

After taking the drug for over two years she reports significant improvement in her quality of life and capacity to accomplish the tasks of everyday living, such as cooking and house cleaning. But her crowning achievement is a return to work. She is now employed 30 hours a week in a "focus-intensive job, doing a great deal of accounting and working with money, problem solving, and multiple product sales." She adds, "I am able to think on my feet, work with many different people during the day, and provide superior customer service. This wasn't possible several years ago." She is even able to ski again! Her remarkable success she attributes to five years of "learning and practicing energy conservation techniques" and just over two years of Ampligen therapy. She credits Ampligen directly for improvements in her memory and, along with specific energy conservation techniques, a shortened recovery time should she overextend herself.

A further endorsement for Ampligen comes from another long time CFS sufferer. Like the first participant, she was diagnosed with CFS over 10 years ago and began Ampligen therapy a little over two years ago. Prior to beginning Ampligen therapy, she also had made some progress toward coping with her illness through a program of therapeutic exercise and energy conservation. Previously she often had to be carried upstairs and used an electric wheelchair when escorting her children to school. Through strategies such as placing a chair mid-way up the stairs to serve as a rest-station and having her children help in the kitchen with chores like "stirring macaroni," she had been able to "get her life back" to some degree.

Currently she is able to walk 2-3 miles without taking a rest break. She can stand for at least an hour, sit up for the entire day, climb two flights of stairs without stopping. No longer does she take naps during the day, or lie down at all. She can run errands, grocery shop, put groceries away, all without resting in-between, do laundry, vacuum the entire house, mop the kitchen, and cook as much as she wants all without symptoms—now the macaroni is "stir, stir, stir, no problem!" Only when she has an infection do the symptoms of CFS reappear. But even then, with the help of antibiotics, she is back to normal activity within 3 to 4 days.

Although reluctant to call her absence of symptoms remission, she feels that she has "attained a normal lifestyle," but is acutely aware that, even with Ampligen and her improved strength levels, she must still take care not do overdo things. However, improvements in cognitive functioning enable her to organize and manage her energy expenditure to best advantage and "do as much activity as any other women with three kids."

Family life also seemed to be positively affected. The most powerful evidence for this came from the spouses. As one husband affirmed, "The saddest part of this disease is that it destroys families. It destroys children. Being able to see his mother get better has given our six-year-old a new spark. You just feel like she has gotten her life back." The other husband also remarked that his wife was "coming back" to him.

CONCLUSION

Whether or not a combination of Ampligen therapy, energy conservation, and therapeutic exercise has brought about a state of remission in these two women, their case histories certainly provide some element of hope that diagnosis of CFS does not necessarily mean the end of an active, healthy and fairly normal life. When one examines the definition of remission, meaning a reduction in the force or intensity of something, or the shortening of a sentence, the changed lives of these women certainly seem to qualify as remission from what must have seemed, for a long time, like a life sentence with no possibility of parole.

REFERENCES

1. Strayer DR, Carter W, Strauss K, Brodsky I, Suhadolnik R, Ablashi D, Henry B, Mitchell WM, Bastein S, Peterson D. Long term improvements in patients with chronic fatigue syndrome treated with Ampligen. *Journal of Chronic Fatigue Syndrome* 1995; 1 (1): 35-53.

2. Racciatti D, Barberia A, Vecchiet J, Pizzigallo E. Clinical and pathogenetical characterization of 238 patients of a chronic fatigue syndrome Italian center. *Journal of Chronic Fatigue Syndrome* 1999; 5 (3/4): 61-70.

3. Suhadolnik RJ, Reichenback NL, Hitzges P, Sobol RW, Peterson DL, Henry B, Ablashi DV, Carter WA, Strayer DR. Upregulation of the 2-5A synthetase/Rnase L antiviral pathway associated with chronic fatigue syndrome. *Clinical Infectious Diseases* 1994; 18: S96-S104.

4. Suhadolnik RJ, Riechenback NL, Sobol RW, Hart R, Peterson DL, Strayer DR, Henry B, Ablashi DB, Gillespie DH, Carter WA. Biochemical defects in the 2-5A synthetase/Rnase L pathway associated with chronic fatigue syndrome with encephalopathy. In: Hyde B, ed., The Clinical and Scientific Basis of Myaligic Encephalomyelitis/Chronic Fatigue Syndrome. The Nightengale Research Foundation, Ottawa, pp. 613-617, 1992.

5. Komaroff AL. A 56-year-old woman with chronic fatigue syndrome. *JAMA* 1997; 278: 1179-1185.

6. Messias DK, Yeager KA, Dibble SL, Dodd MJ. Patient's perspectives of fatigue while undergoing chemotherapy. *Oncology Nursing Forum* 1997; 24 (1): 43-48.

7. Ream E, Richardson A. Fatigue in patients with cancer and chronic obstructive airways disease: a phenomenological enquiry. *International Journal of Nursing Studies* 1997; 34 (1): 44-53.

8. Snell CR, Stevens SR. Opening the envelope. *The CFIDS Chronicle* 1998; 11 (2): 12-13.